S0-ARL-848

UNDERSTANDING CHEST RADIOGRAPHS

UNDERSTANDING CHEST RADIOGRAPHS

Joseph L. Rau, Jr. M.A., R.R.T.
Douglas J. Pearce, B.S., R.R.T.

Multi-Media Publishing, inc.
Denver, Colorado

©Copyright 1984 by Multi-Media Publishing, Inc., Denver, Colorado
First Edition

All rights reserved. No part of this book may be reproduced in any form or by any means without permission in writing from the publisher.

Printed in the United States of America

MULTI-MEDIA PUBLISHING, INC., BOOK DIVISION
1393 S. INCA STREET, DENVER, COLORADO 80223

Library of Congress Cataloging in Publication Data

Rau, Joseph L.
    Understanding chest radiographs.

    Bibliography: p.
    Includes index.
    1. Chest—Radiography.   2. Chest—Diseases—Diagnosis.
3. Diagnosis, Radioscopic. I. Pearce, Douglas J.,
1953-   . II. Title. [DNLM: 1. Thoracic radiography.
WF 975 R239u]
RC941.R28 1984   617'.5407572   83-62443
ISBN 0-940122-11-1

MMP/BC/BC 9 8 7 6 5 4 3 2 1

Dedication

To Agnes, Mary Agnes, and Joseph III. J.L.R., Jr.
To my parents and Barbara. D.J.P.

About the Authors

Joseph L. Rau, Jr. is an Assistant Professor in the Department of Respiratory Therapy at Georgia State University in Atlanta, Georgia, where he has held a faculty position since 1974. He has been involved with both lecture courses and clinical instruction in the basic modes of respiratory care, pharmacology, critical care, and patient assessment. Between 1976 and 1978 he held an HEW grant to develop computer instruction software for respiratory care. He was given the Alumni Distinguished Professor Award in the College of Health Sciences at Georgia State University for teaching, research and professional service in 1976. In 1977, he received the Warner-Chilcott Literary Award for his *Respiratory Care* publication on computer-assisted instruction. He has published a number of articles on respiratory care, and is a charter member of the Georgia State Chapter of Alpha Eta Honor Society, the national scholarship society for health sciences. He is currently completing a doctoral degree in educational research and measurement, and is a registered respiratory therapist.

Douglas J. Pearce held the position of Clinical Consultant for the Department of Respiratory Care at Piedmont Hospital, Atlanta, Georgia. In that position, he had the responsibility for evaluating patients' respiratory status and planning their respiratory care. He is currently pursuing a M.D. at the Medical College of Georgia, Augusta, Georgia. He has been involved in the field of respiratory care in various clinical capacities since 1974, both in Florida and Georgia.

He has also been active in a number of professionally related organizations, including the American Lung Association, Georgia Lung Association, the Atlanta Lung Association, and is a member of the American Association for Respiratory Therapy, as well as the Georgia Society for Respiratory Therapy. He is a registered respiratory theraptist.

Preface

This text is intended to be a concise resource on interpreting chest radiographs. The goal is to provide the reader with the basis for understanding chest radiographs in an applied clinical setting, not as a radiologist, but as a clinician involved in critical and respiratory care. The specific target reader is the nonphysician clinical practitioner, for example, the respiratory therapist, critical care nurse, nurse practitioner, or pulmonary physician's assistant. The technical aspects of producing radiographs are discussed only minimally and to the extent necessary to enhance the clinical understanding of chest radiographs.

Although prior knowledge of radiology is not assumed, the text will be more useful if the reader has a basic, but sound understanding of thoracic anatomy. In addition, a minimal familiarity with the specific disease processes mentioned and the thoracic changes produced will facilitate understanding of the radiographic appearance of those processes. Finally, it would be helpful to know commonly employed supportive and monitoring measures with critical care patients, in order to recognize their appearance on a radiograph. Examples of these measures include endotracheal tubes, electrocardiogram leads, and Swan-Ganz catheters.

The text is divided into two major sections. Part One presents the principles of interpreting chest radiographs, including the physics of x-rays, standard and specialized chest radiographic techniques, anatomical findings, method of inspection, and clinical findings such as the silhouette sign and the air bronchogram. Lung perfusion and ventilation scans are briefly discussed. In Part Two these principles are applied to the interpretation of chest radiographs in a series of cases. The objectives of Part Two are twofold: first, to give the reader *practice* in applying the principles given in Part One; and second, to present the *classic* radiologic appearances of typical chest abnormalities, including pneumothorax, chest tubes, pneumonias, pulmonary masses, chest traumas and chronic pulmonary disease entities. The cases in Part Two were chosen because they present clearly the classic appearance of chest abnormalities and demonstrate the need for their recognition and correct interpretation by practitioners. The sequence of the contents in Part Two is based, primarily, on the importance of correctly recognizing certain conditions. The identification of endotracheal tubes and their proper positioning is followed by several cases of pneumothorax, including a case of chest trauma with rib fractures. Cases showing a variety of pulmonary infiltrates, such as atelectasis, pneumonia, adult respiratory distress syndrome (ARDS) and congestive heart failure, are then presented. Chronic pulmonary diseases are exemplified by chronic obstructive pulmonary disease (COPD), miliary tuberculosis and cylindrical bronchiectasis. Several examples of pulmonary masses, from nodule to metastatic carcinoma, are given. Cases illustrating pulmonary embolism with accompanying lung scans, cystic fibrosis, pneumoconiosis, histoplasmosis, lung abscess and pleural effusion, and subdiaphragmatic air are presented as a sequence of radiographs in decreasing order of importance for the critical care practitioner. A multiple gunshot victim case is offered for practice and self-assessment. Finally, a table summarizing chest radiographic signs and common abnormalities, and a glossary of selected radiographic and related terms are provided.

Acknowledgments

The material contained in this text was produced in cooperation with the Department of Respiratory Therapy at Georgia State University and the Departments of Respiratory Care and Radiology at Piedmont Hospital in Atlanta, Georgia. Without the willingness of these departments to allow access to radiographs and other materials, the text would not have been possible. We are grateful to the following clinicians for reviewing the text and offering numerous suggestions for improvements: Barbara Krueger, R.R.T., of Piedmont Hospital, Atlanta, Georgia and Robert J. Bachmann, R.R.T., H. Bruce Bray, R.R.T., Albert K. Blackwelder, R.R.T., and Gerald W. Staton, Jr., M.D., all of Crawford W. Long Memorial Hospital, Atlanta, Georgia. In addition, we are grateful to William A. Hopkins, M.D., Medical Director of the Department of Respiratory Therapy at Georgia State University, who shared his considerable experience in interpreting some of the x-ray films. The recommendations of the publisher's reviewer, Bruce Broswick, R.R.T., were of considerable benefit to the authors. We wish also to thank Elizabeth Davis and Leigh Walling for patiently bearing the burden of typing several drafts of the manuscript. Finally, we wish to thank each other for mutual encouragement in completing this task.

—Joseph L. Rau, Jr.
Douglas J. Pearce

Table of Contents

Part One

Introduction to the Basic Principles of Chest Radiology

RADIATION PHYSICS

"Our intellectual careers begin to bud in the incessant 'What?' and 'Why?' of childhood. They flower only if we are willing, or constrained, to learn how to learn. They bring forth fruit only after the discovery that, if we really would master the answers, we somehow have to find them out ourselves."

B.J.F. Lonergan
Insight: A Study of Human Understanding, 1957

In 1895, Wilhelm Roentgen, a German physicist, first noticed that by passing an experimental ray through his wife's hand he could produce a shadow image of her hand bones on photographic film *(Fig. 1-1)*. Roentgen called the unknown rays he had discovered "x-rays." In honor of Roentgen's discovery, x-ray films are also sometimes called roentgenograms. However, the actual technical term for an exposed x-ray film is **radiograph.**

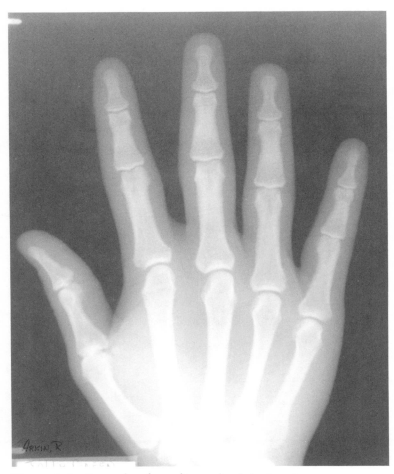

Figure 1-1. Example of a radiograph of the hand.

X-rays are produced by the impact of high velocity electrons from a cathode onto a target made of suitable metal (*Fig. 1-2A*). These rays can penetrate solids and produce a shadow image of the solid when they strike a plate of film. X-rays are waves and, as such, exhibit the properties common to all waves: wavelength (lambda—λ), frequency (f) or cycles per unit time, and velocity (v). Velocity is constant (the speed of light); therefore, the wavelength of a given wave decreases if the frequency increases (*see* Fig. 1-2B). Doubling the frequency decreases the wavelength by half. As waves, x-rays are part of the electromagnetic spectrum. X-rays have a shorter wavelength, but a higher frequency, than visible or ultraviolet light, and have a much higher frequency than radio or television waves (*Fig. 1-2C*).

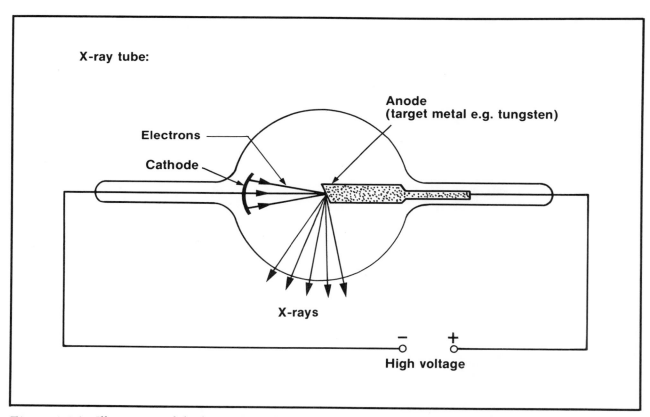

Figure 1-2A. Illustration of the basic principle in producing x-radiation.

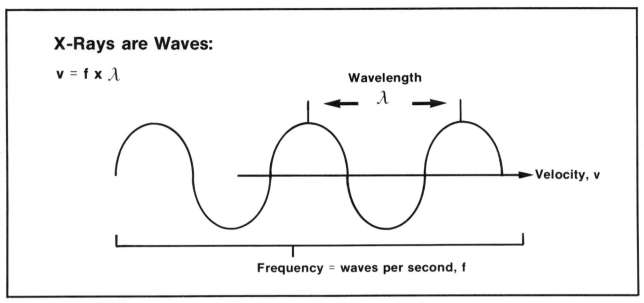

Figure 1-2B. Relationship between wavelength and wave frequency: wavelength decreases if frequency increases.

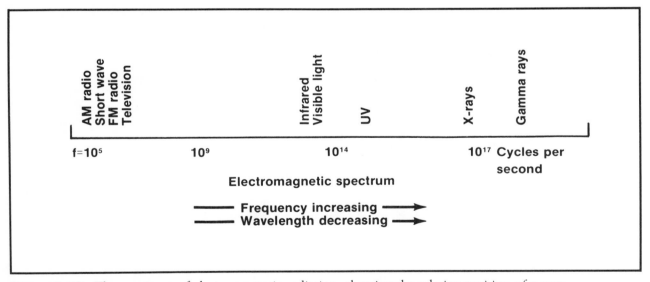

Figure 1-2C. The spectrum of electromagnetic radiation, showing the relative position of x-rays.

The interaction between x-rays and human tissue is based on the energy of x-rays. This energy equals the frequency multiplied by a constant (h = 6.63×10^{-34} Joule seconds), which is called Planck's constant in honor of the German physicist, Max Planck, who quantified the energy-frequency relationship. Higher frequencies yield higher amounts of energy, as seen by the equation, $E = h \times f$, where h is Planck's constant, f is frequency, and E equals energy (Fig. 1-3). X-rays have enough energy to pass through less dense atoms (tissue, skin, air), but are absorbed by heavier atoms (bone, metal clips), producing the dark, exposed areas and light, unexposed areas on radiographs. For example, lung fields full of air and soft tissue appear dark, whereas bone appears white.

The relative order of density from least dense (dark on the radiograph*) to most dense (light or white on the radiograph) is gas, fat, water, bone and metal.

Unfortunately, the energy of x-rays that allows for the penetration of substances and the exposure of film can also ionize and cause radiation effects; therefore, exposure to such rays should be limited.

The images seen on chest radiographs result from the differences in densities of materials in the body. Dense materials absorb *more* x-rays, and less dense materials absorb *less* x-rays. X-rays pass through the body to expose the film. Dense material, such as bone or a metal clip, absorbs much of the x-ray and leaves the film relatively unexposed. The shadow of such dense material shows up as white or gray-white on the radiograph when it is developed. Large, relatively dense organs, such as the heart, also appear whitish on the radiograph. Skin and soft tissue are not as dense as bone and appear more translucent, but they are still whitish.

Energy of x-rays affects their interaction with human tissue.

Energy = h x f (h = Planck's constant, f = frequency)

Dense material (bone) — absorbs more x-rays — film unexposed (white or gray-white)

Less dense material (lungs) — absorbs less x-rays — film exposed (black or dark gray)

Relative Order of Radiographic Densities (least dense to most dense)

- **Gas—present in lungs, stomach, intestines**
- **Fat—surrounds kidney; present along the abdominal wall and other organs**
- **Water—same density as heart and blood vessels**
- **Bone—more dense than other tissues**
- **Metal—foreign objects, prosthesis, contrast media**

Ionizing radiation can cause biological damage; exposure should be limited.

Figure 1-3. Summary of the physical basis for the energy of x-rays and its effects.

---

*A note on the terminology used in this text may help prevent confusion or misunderstanding. In the clinical setting, practitioners often speak of a radiograph as an x-ray. Technically, an x-ray is a form of electromagnetic radiation, not the exposed and developed film that the practitioner examines; therefore, throughout this text the term "x-ray" will be used to mean the actual x-ray waves. The exposed film that the practitioner views will be called a **radiograph.** Other terms often used in discussing radiographs are "projection" and "position." **Projection** refers to the path of an x-ray beam as it enters and exits the body. For example, a posteroanterior projection means that the beam enters the back and exits the front of the chest. **Position** refers to the specific body position, such as supine, erect, Fowler's, and so forth.

In addition to the basic production and appearance of radiographs, a number of descriptive terms and concepts are used in conjunction with radiographs and are important for the clinical understanding of the films. These terms and concepts include the various projections and positions used with patients when the radiograph is produced, such as posteroanterior versus lateral, and the techniques that are employed to enhance the visualization of the chest, such as bronchography and tomography. Each of these concepts and the corresponding terminology are discussed and illustrated in the following sections. In addition, a glossary is included at the end of the book as a reference for terms that are commonly encountered in discussions of radiographs.

(Note: Technically, translucent means transparent to light; because x-rays and not visible light are being used, the corresponding term is radiolucent, i.e., more transparent to x-radiation.) The air-filled lungs are the least dense of the chest components that have been mentioned. They appear dark on a radiograph. There is minimal absorption of the x-rays, which reach the film, expose it, and produce varying darknesses after development. Lung tissue does have some density, and so-called tissue markings can be distinguished with careful inspection. These tissue markings appear as short, whitish streaks and lines throughout the area of the lung fields. In fact, a pneumothorax, which involves partial or complete lung collapse and air in the pleural space, can be recognized by clear radiolucency and *absence* of tissue markings. Remember that air is less dense than tissue. In addition, a collapsed lung appears as *more* densely compacted with a visible border. Ease of recognition is directly proportional to the size of the pneumothorax. Several cases of pneumothorax are presented in Part Two to help the practitioner to identify this abnormality.

The *absolute* degree of whiteness or darkness in a chest radiograph is a function of both density in the chest, and intensity and degree of exposure to x-rays. While the heart may appear white on one radiograph, the same heart may be less white or more radiolucent on another film with more exposure. The analogy relates to ordinary light-sensitive film, which can be underexposed or overexposed. The same is true for film that is exposed to x-rays. The principal guideline behind interpreting chest radiographs is this: evaluate darkness and lightness of an area or organ *in relation to* the degree of darkness and lightness of other areas having a known relative density. For example, if the lung fields are dark and lack tissue markings, the heart and other areas should be checked. If the heart, which is denser in relation to lung fields, is also darker than expected, the entire film may be overexposed. If so, there is no absolute loss of tissue in the lung. Specific guidelines for evaluating the relative degree of exposure for a given film are presented in Part One under the heading "Method of Inspecting the Chest Radiograph." Distinctions of relative densities form the basis for clinically interpreting the appearance of a chest radiograph and for evaluating the technical quality of the radiograph.

STANDARD POSITIONS AND TECHNIQUES OF CHEST RADIOGRAPHY

The Posteroanterior (PA) Position

The standard position for obtaining a routine, adult chest radiograph is the posteroanterior (PA), with the patient standing upright. In this position (*Fig. 1-4*), the front of the patient's chest is placed against the film, and the x-ray source is 72 in. (6 ft.) from the film. The shoulders are rotated forward to touch the film, ensuring that the scapulae (shoulder blades) do not obscure a portion of the lung field. The radiograph is usually taken with the patient in full inspiration, lowering the diaphragm to the ninth to eleventh ribs posteriorly. Expiratory radiographs are also taken to demonstrate diaphragmatic excursion and the symmetry or asymmetry of such excursion. Expiratory chest radiographs are beneficial in diagnosing the pathology of a pneumothorax, to be discussed later.

There are a number of advantages to obtaining an upright PA radiograph in addition to being able to rotate the scapulae out of the lung fields. With the six-foot distance between the x-ray tube and the film, magnification is reduced and the sharpness of the image created by the x-ray beam is improved. Because the heart occupies the front half of the thorax, placing the front of the chest against the film and having the x-ray beam strike from behind reduces the magnification of the heart (*Fig. 1-10*). The diaphragm is also lower in an upright position than in a recumbent position. Fluid, if present, will gravitate to dependent portions of the lung or chest, and may be more easily seen. One of the most significant values of taking upright chest radiographs is that air-fluid levels are readily identifiable.

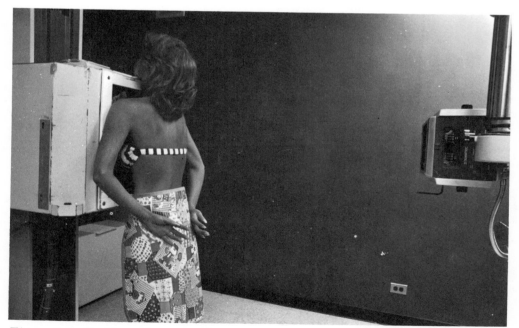

Figure 1-4. Position of a patient for a posteroanterior (PA), upright chest radiograph.

A very real, but often overlooked advantage of the PA projection is the fact that it presents the standard anatomical position. In the PA upright position, the chest will be seen as it is usually described anatomically. For the beginning student, this is a great aid in evaluating the relationships of organs, as well as in identifying the initially unfamiliar appearance of anatomical landmarks on a radiograph.

In viewing a PA radiograph, the practitioner should imagine looking at the patient from the front (the patient's left side on the viewer's right).

Imagine that the x-ray is a beam of light hitting the patient from behind, passing through and illuminating the chest contents for the viewer, who is standing in front of the patient. When the radiograph is placed on a view box, the left side of the chest is on the right side of the viewer and is usually indicated by a large L. If the person does not have **situs inversus** (reversal of internal thoracic organs), the aortic arch will appear on the left and the predominant left ventricle will be on the left side of the cardiac shadow.

Figure 1-5 is an example of an actual postero-anterior chest radiograph. As much as possible, the practitioner should check each chest radiograph for indications of the patient's position. The most obvious and helpful indicator is the radiologist's report, but several other aspects of the radiograph itself should be noted. First, in a PA radiograph the scapulae are rotated out of the chest area as much as possible. Recall that the shoulders are brought forward to touch the film, with the patient's chest against the film. This will often not be the case in an anteroposterior (AP) radiograph since patients chosen for AP films may be unable to adequately rotate their scapulae or to cooperate in general because of their condition. Consequently, the scapulae will often be visible in an AP radiograph. Second, the upright position can be verified by the air-fluid line in the stomach, if such a line is visible. Gravity keeps an air-fluid line parallel to the floor; therefore, a horizontal line indicates that a patient was upright when the radiograph was taken.

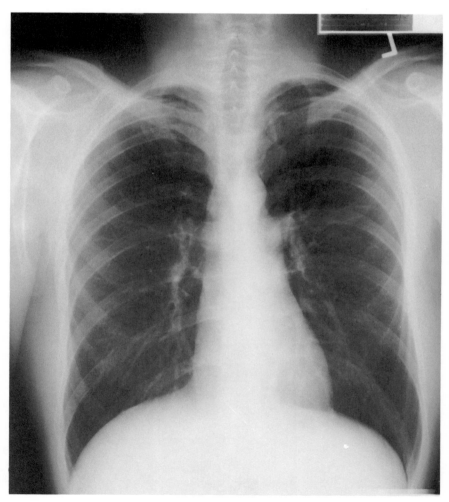

Figure 1-5. Example of a PA chest radiograph of an adult patient.

The Lateral Position

The PA radiograph is complemented by the lateral upright radiograph, in which the patient's side is placed against the film. In a lateral upright film, the patient usually stands with arms raised over the head to prevent the arms from obscuring or overlying the thorax (*Fig. 1-6*). In a frontal (PA) radiograph, the heart and the anteroposterior slope of the diaphragm obscure much of the space in the chest. The lateral position allows the viewer to see behind the heart and diaphragmatic dome. Also, the lateral radiograph can be put together with a PA radiograph of the same chest (in the mind of the viewer) to determine the three-dimensional position of organs or abnormal densities. This allows the clinician to localize a point within the thorax. Tracheostomy tubes, for example, are well defined in lateral radiographs (*see Figures 2-7 and 2-8*). A left lateral radiograph is usually obtained (left side of the patient against the film) to reduce heart magnification. (The heart occupies more of the left chest.) However, if an abnormality is known to be present in the chest, the side that brings the abnormality closest to the film is placed against the film. Thus, a right-sided density or lesion is better evaluated with a right lateral radiograph. Also, it should be noted that one cannot always visualize a density on a lateral film that may be seen well on the corresponding PA film.

When looking at a lateral film, the viewer should try to distinguish the right and left hemidiaphragms. Usually, the right hemidiaphragm is higher than the left. This can be confirmed in an individual if the corresponding PA film is available. In the lateral radiograph, the right hemidiaphragm is usually *above* the left, although the two borders may cross as the diaphragm slopes toward the back of the thorax. Because the heart is in physical contact with the left diaphragm, visualization of the left diaphragm ends at the cardiac shadow. In contrast, the dome of the right diaphragm may be seen extending anteriorly *beyond* the cardiac shadow.

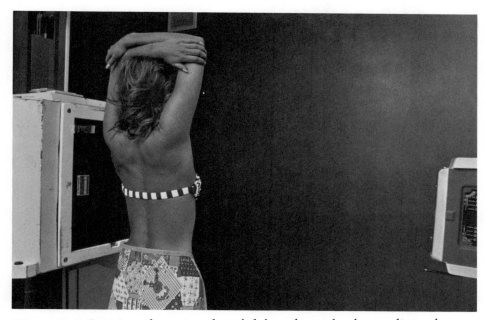

Figure 1-6. Position of a patient for a left lateral upright chest radiograph.

Figure 1-7 is an example of a lateral radiograph. Again, a horizontal air-fluid line in the stomach often verifies the upright position. Unfortunately, *Figure 1-7* does not show any fluid line below the diaphragm. Details of the normal anatomy that should be found in a lateral radiograph are given in *Figures 1-25 through 1-27.*

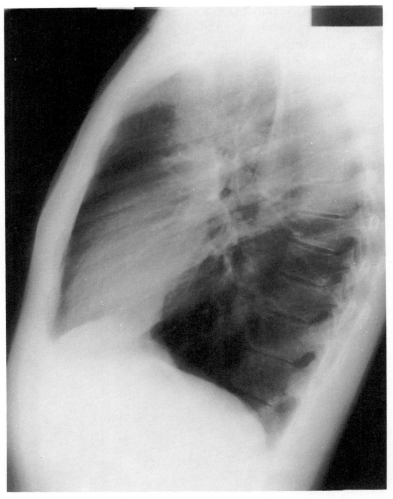

Figure 1-7. Example of a left lateral upright chest radiograph in an adult patient.

The Anteroposterior (AP) Position

When the patient is debilitated, immobilized, or too young to cooperate with the PA procedure, or when a posterior abnormality is to be viewed, an anteroposterior radiograph can be taken. It may be taken with a portable unit or taken in the radiology department (*Fig. 1-8*). The film is placed behind the patient's back, with the x-ray source usually 36 to 40 inches from the film when a portable unit is used. Due to physical constraints, this distance is often necessary in acutely ill or debilitated patients requiring a portable radiographic procedure. Actually, a 72 in. distance from x-ray tube to film is preferred whenever possible on an AP radiograph to improve the sharpness of the image. There may be distortion, greater coarseness and less resolution with an AP radiograph. Because the patient chosen for an AP procedure is often debilitated, acutely ill or very young, it may not be possible to obtain good inspiratory radiographs or symmetrical chest positions. Artifactual shadows from ventilator tubing, intravenous lines or other indwelling lines will often be present.

In the representative chest AP radiograph depicted in *Figure 1-9*, the larger appearance of the cardiac shadow is caused by the magnification previously mentioned and further illustrated in *Figure 1-10*. *Figure 1-9* also shows the presence of the scapulae, which usually are not rotated out of view in this position.

The positioning of the body determines how close to the x-ray film a given organ, such as the heart, may be. Because the heart occupies the anterior portion of the chest in an AP radiograph, the heart is farther away from the film and, subsequently, often appears enlarged. As seen in *Figure 1-10*, the closer the heart is to the film, the smaller the shadow (image) that is produced. It is not unusual to see the cardiac shadow slightly enlarged in an AP projection (*Fig. 1-10*). To properly evaluate apparent enlargements, it is important to know the patient's position when the radiograph was taken.

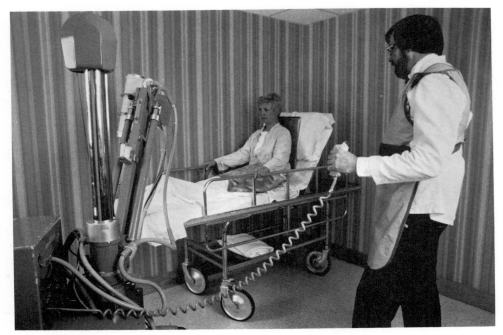

Figure 1-8. Position of a patient for an anteroposterior (AP) chest radiograph.

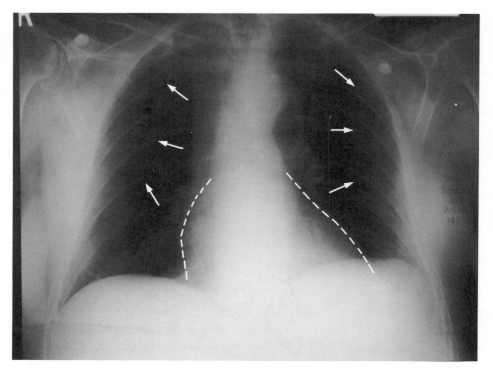

Figure 1-9. Example of an AP chest radiograph. The cardiac shadow (outline) appears larger than in a PA radiograph. Scapulae (arrows) are shown in the film.

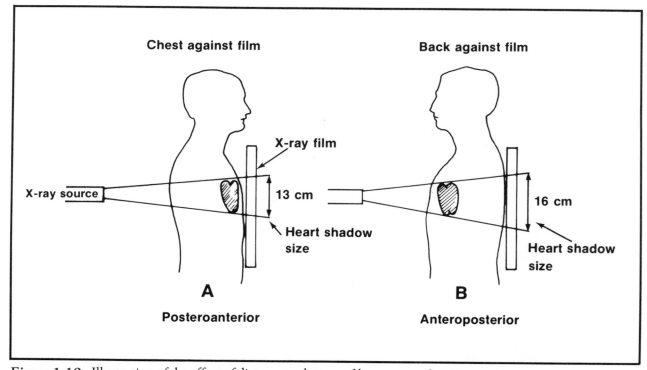

Figure 1-10. Illustration of the effect of distance to the x-ray film on magnification.

The Oblique Position

The oblique position *(Fig. 1-11)* is another useful technique that enables the practitioner to see behind and around overlying chest structures. The oblique position is particularly helpful in avoiding the radiographic superimposition of bilateral abnormalities that might occur in a lateral radiograph. The terms **right oblique** and **left oblique** refer to positions in which the right and left shoulders are rotated in relation to the surface of the x-ray film. By so turning the patient, the angle at which the x-ray passes through the chest is shifted, and previously superimposed shadows of organs or lesions are spread apart. This displacement phenomenon is termed **parallax.** The terminology of oblique positions is straightforward: the oblique position coincides with the part of the patient that is closest to the x-ray film. For example, a right anterior oblique radiograph is taken with the patient's right front against the film, at an angle of approximately 45 degrees *(Fig. 1-11)*. In the right posterior oblique position, the right side of the patient's back is against the film.

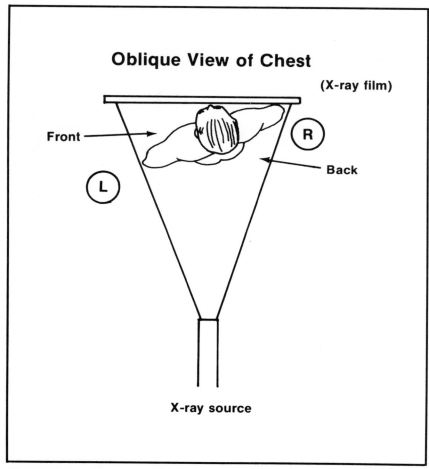

Oblique View of Chest

(X-ray film)

Front

R

Back

L

X-ray source

Figure 1-11. Position of the patient for an oblique chest radiograph. A right anterior oblique radiograph is obtained in this position.

Figure 1-12 is a representative radiograph illustrating the oblique position. Contrast media has been used to outline the esophagus, allowing the viewer to see the relative shift in the mediastinal structures. It may be easiest to imagine looking diagonally through the chest, somewhere between a straight frontal and a straight lateral projection. The trachea, esophagus, vertebrae and heart are no longer superimposed as in a PA chest radiograph. Instead, each of these structures has been spread out by the oblique angle, permitting greater ease in seeing around the organs involved.

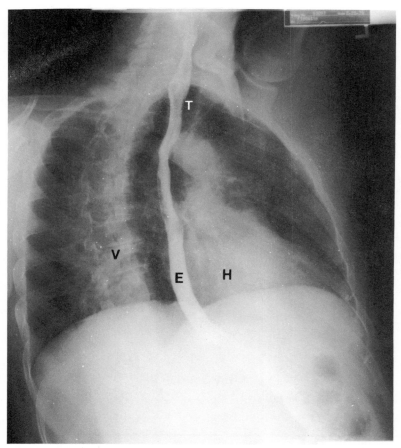

Figure 1-12. Example of a chest radiograph taken in the oblique position. This particular radiograph is of a right anterior oblique position. Trachea (T), esophagus (E), vertebrae (V), and heart (H) are spread out by the oblique angle.

The Lordotic Position

Originally, the lordotic chest radiograph was achieved by having the patient lean backward with the back arched, projecting the clavicles above the lung field and causing the anterior and posterior ribs to be parallel. It is easier, however, to lower the x-ray tube than to have the patient arch backward *(Fig. 1-13)*. A lordotic chest radiograph is helpful in giving a clearer view of the upper lung fields, which are obscured by bony structures (clavicle, first and second ribs) in the PA position.

The clavicles are projected upward and the ribs are made parallel to the angle of the x-ray beam. As a result, the clavicles do not obstruct the view of the apex, and the posterior and anterior portions of the ribs are superimposed, presenting a straight appearance and further helping to clear the upper lung area.

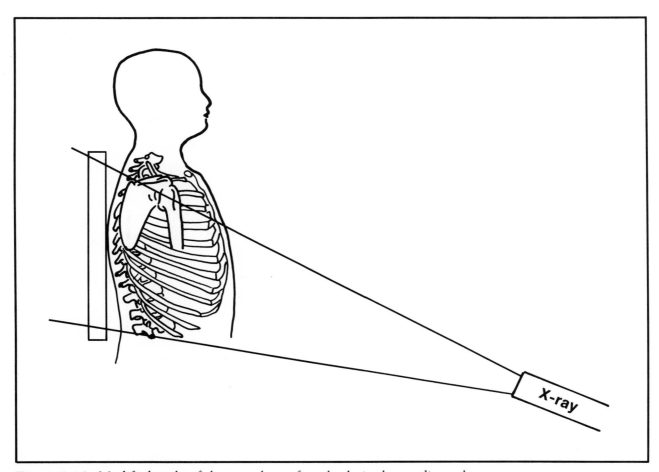

Figure 1-13. Modified angle of the x-ray beam for a lordotic chest radiograph.

The lordotic position also has the effect of moving an anterior density up and a posterior density down (*Fig. 1-14*). This can be more easily understood by imagining someone arching backward in lordosis: the front of the chest moves up and the back moves down. This effect is the same as crouching down and looking up toward the chest. Although an anterior and a posterior point are superimposed on a straight frontal position, they can be separated by changing the x-ray beam angle.

Figure 1-15 is a radiograph taken in the lordotic position. The ribs appear differently, being much flatter and parallel to each other. The clavicles are very high and can be seen above the apices. Because the air-fluid level in the stomach is horizontal, it is safe to assume that the radiograph was taken with the patient in an upright position. Most lordotic radiographs are AP.

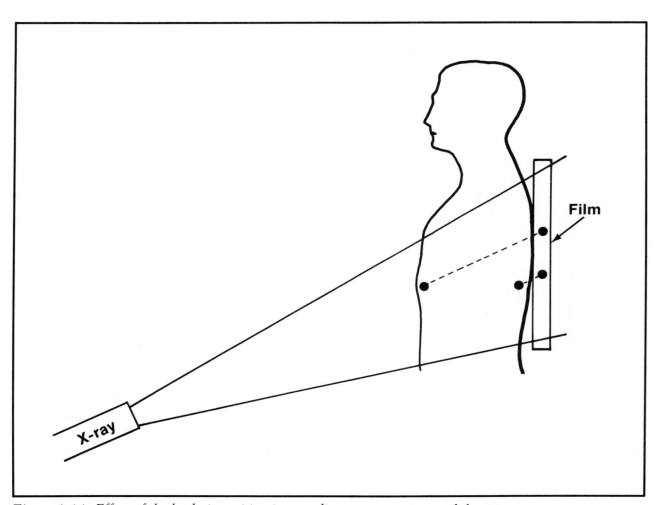

Figure 1-14. Effect of the lordotic position in spreading apart superimposed densities.

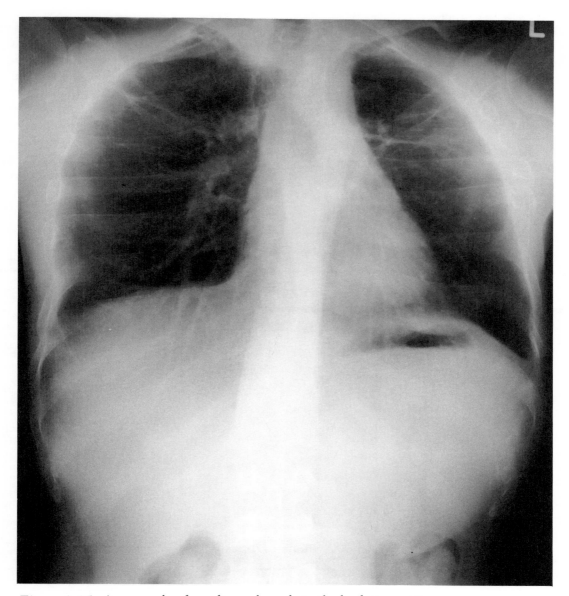

Figure 1-15. An example of a radiograph made in the lordotic position.

Conventional Tomography

Tomography is a procedure that is helpful in evaluating lesions, densities and/or other abnormalities, such as cavities in the chest. A tomogram is made by simultaneously moving the x-ray source and the film plate, usually by a connecting arm, so that the axis of rotation corresponds to a certain depth within the patient's chest (Fig. 1-16). As a result, only one plane is focused on the radiograph. By changing the depth at which this plane of focus occurs, successive slices can be taken through any chest abnormality. This procedure does not give a sharper image than PA or AP techniques, but it does give better visualization of a site by selectively blurring other areas.

Although several types of x-ray tube motions are possible with modern tomographic equipment (linear, circular, elliptical, etc.), chest tomography usually employs linear motion. Conventional chest tomography is different from computed tomography, a procedure involving computer processing of x-rays to generate a cross-sectional image.

Tomograms of the chest are very useful for evaluating areas of the pulmonary parenchyma and mediastinum. An AP projection is usually used, with the patient in a supine position. A parenchymal density or abnormality can be examined with regard to its inner appearance (calcium, cavitation, air bronchogram), outer appearance (border definition and contour, shape), and surrounding area (satellite nodules, connected vessels). Tomograms of the hilar region can show normal blood vessels, masses, nodes, calcification, bronchial compression and endobronchial lesions. Tomography of either parenchymal or hilar nodules is especially useful in evaluating suspected carcinoma.

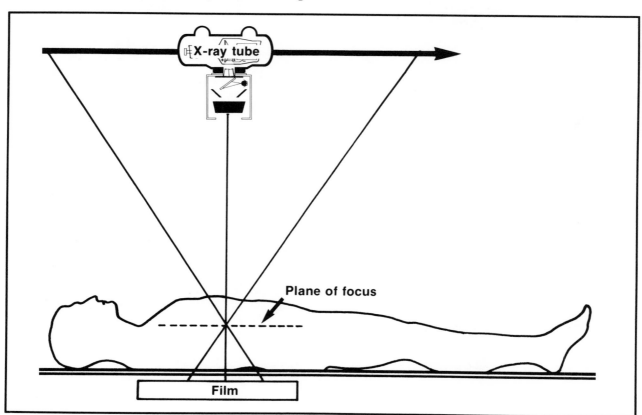

Figure 1-16. Illustration of the principle employed in creating a tomogram.

Part of a conventional tomogram series is shown in *Figure 1-17*, illustrating the technique's typical blurred appearance. The series in *Figure 1-17* was obtained to evaluate a large right upper lobe density that appeared in a PA radiograph. Going clockwise and starting in the upper left corner, four successively deeper slices of the density were taken. The inner appearance differentiates this density as a solid mass, not a cavity. This particular case, in which tomograms were used as an adjunct to the PA chest radiograph, is discussed further in Part Two, the section entitled "Large Right Upper Lobe Mass."

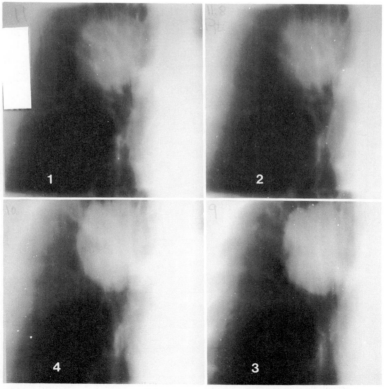

Figure 1-17. A series of four tomograms used to visualize a right upper lobe density.

Bronchography

Through the use of instilled contrast medium, such as Dionosil, the tracheobronchial tree can be readily seen (*Fig. 1-18*). The **bronchogram** (the term used for a radiograph obtained in this way) is useful in diagnosing bronchogenic carcinoma, lesions of the tracheobronchial tree, and congenital abnormalities of the lung. It is used most often to diagnose deterioration of airways caused by the long-term effects of chronic pulmonary disease, such as bronchiectasis. A bronchogram is often performed to map portions of a diseased lung prior to surgery, or to decide if surgery should be performed, although the frequency of this technique seems to be declining. The contrast material provides a very clear outline of the trachea, carina, right and left main stem bronchi, bronchiolar branching and segmental bronchioles. This technique is helpful for the beginning student who has difficulty in seeing the tracheobronchial structure in a normal PA radiograph.

A lateral bronchogram is shown in *Figure 1-19*. The PA and lateral bronchogram can be useful in learning the segmental and lobar anatomy of the lung. By comparing the two, the beginner gets a sense of the lung's three-dimensional positioning. Those who are unfamiliar with the relative positioning of the tracheobronchial tree in PA and lateral radiographs should study *Figures 1-18 and 1-19* carefully.

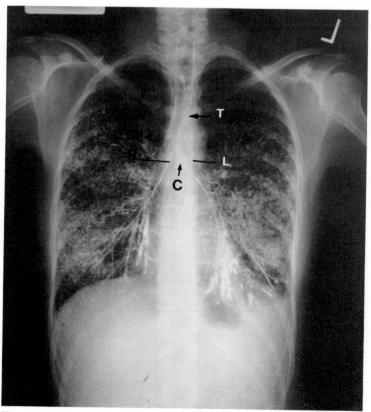

Figure 1-18. An example of an adult bronchogram taken with a PA projection. Trachea (T), carina (C), right (R) and left (L) main stem bronchi are clearly shown.

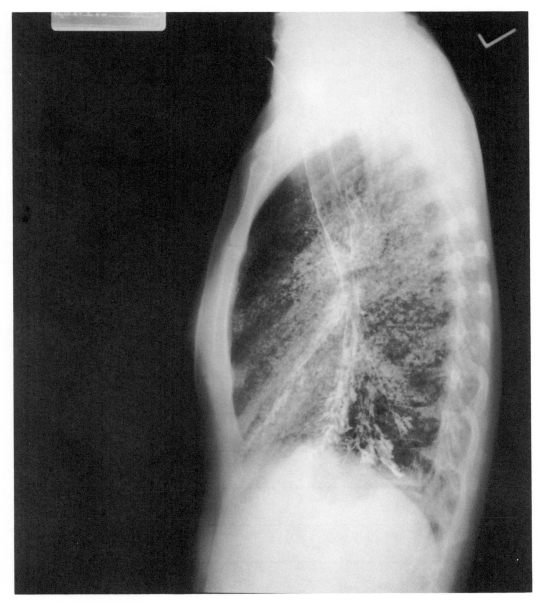

Figure 1-19. An example of a bronchogram with a lateral projection.

Lateral Decubitus Position

Another technique used in chest radiography is the lateral decubitus position, in which the patient lies on either the right side (right lateral decubitus) or the left side (left lateral decubitus) when the radiograph is made, rather than standing upright as usual. The position required in taking a left lateral decubitus radiograph is shown in *Figure 1-20*. The naming of decubitus radiographs is determined by the side that is placed down: a left lateral decubitus radiograph means that the left side is down. *Figure 1-21* is a left lateral decubitus radiograph in which the right, or upper side, is clearly marked. Arrows point to a line of fluid in the left pleural space, now accumulating along the downward edge of the left lung, caused by the dependent position of the patient. This position can be further verified by the shifted air-fluid level of the stomach (arrowhead). The lateral decubitus position is often useful in revealing a suspected or known pleural fluid that cannot be seen easily in a PA radiograph. The pleural effusion, which is more thinly spread out in upright or even semi-reclining AP radiographs, collects in a dependent position, allowing it to be seen in *Figure 1-21*.

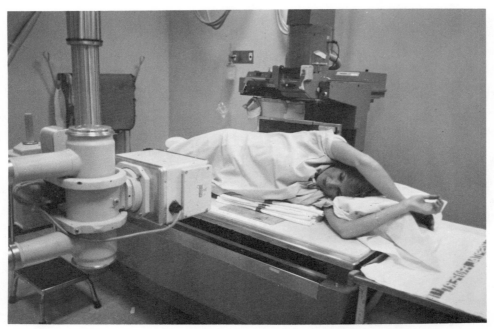

Figure 1-20. Position of the patient for a left lateral decubitus radiograph.

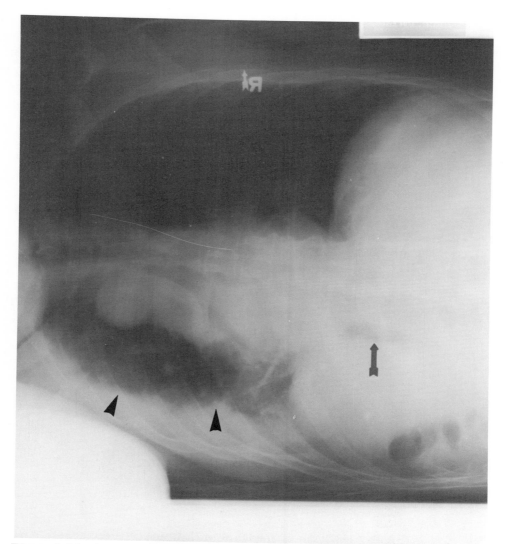

Figure 1-21. An example of a left lateral decubitus chest radiograph showing pleural effusion (two arrowheads on the left). Note the shifted air-fluid level in the stomach (arrow).

NORMAL ANATOMY SEEN IN CHEST RADIOGRAPHS

Before using a radiograph to detect chest abnormalities, it is important to know the normal chest anatomy that one can expect to see. A normal PA chest radiograph is shown in *Figure 1-22*.

In *Figure 1-23*, the following shadows are outlined and labeled (right and left refer to the right and left sides of the patient's chest, not the viewer's right and left):

A—diaphragm

B—costophrenic angles

C—left ventricle (This may be the right ventricle in infants, which predominates.)

D—the right atrium

E—the right hilum*

F—the left hilum

G—the aortic arch or knob

H—area of the superior vena cava

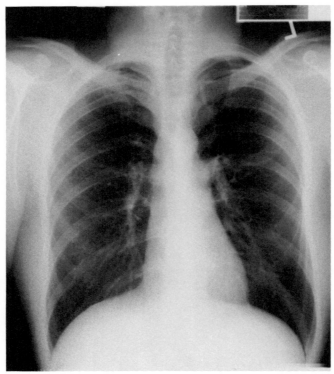

Figure 1-22. An example of a standard PA chest radiograph.

*The term hilum means a "trifle" or "least" in Latin; used in describing the lung, it refers to the origin of the pulmonary arteries and the area where the veins return to the heart. Because these vessels are least spread out or diffused at this point, they create visible densities. The left hilum is usually an interspace higher than the right, assuming that the patient's position is straight. Diagnostically, a lowered left hilum may indicate left lower lobe atelectasis. Thus the relative positioning of the right and left hilar shadows is very informative.

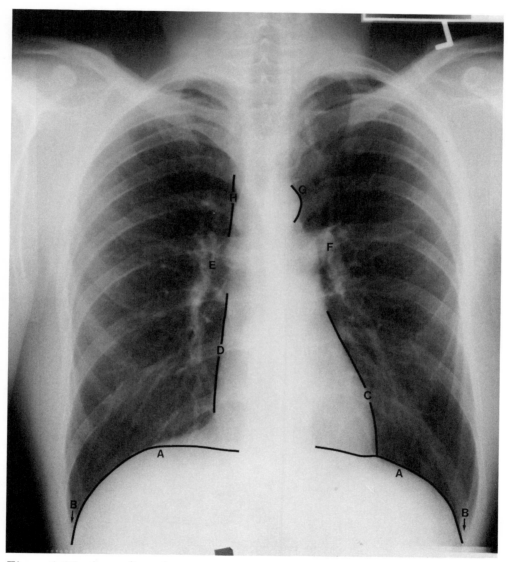

Figure 1-23. An outline of some important anatomical structures usually seen in a PA chest radiograph. (See the text for identifications.)

Figure 1-24 outlines other important landmarks that can be seen in a chest radiograph, as follows:

A—the trachea

B—the main carina or branching point of the right and left main stem bronchi. This site is extremely important and is sometimes difficult to see in the chest radiograph of a patient with an endotracheal tube, the position of which must be evaluated.

C—the clavicles (outlined) along with the first rib from posterior to anterior. The ribs are numbered on the anterior portion. The posterior part of each rib, where it joins a thoracic vertebra, is the most superior part of the rib. They should be traced visually back to their posterior attachments. The anterior and posterior levels of the ribs are very different, and both will be referred to when pointing out chest abnormalities.

D—several of the vertebral bodies (outlined)

E—the scapula on the right side (indicated)

Finally, the cardiothoracic ratio (C-T ratio) is outlined and should be checked. The usual ratio of maximal cardiac width to the total width of the thorax, as measured at the diaphragm level, is less than 50 percent in adults (less than 60 percent in infants). This determination is, of course, less accurate in AP radiographs because of the magnification problem.

In the cases presented in this text, the frequent use of anatomical landmarks seen on chest radiographs, such as rib levels, intercostal spaces and clavicles, will help localize the position of abnormalities.

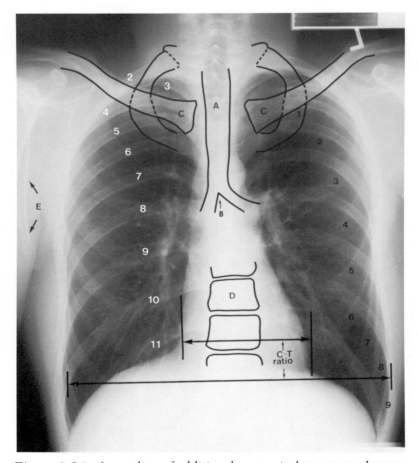

Figure 1-24. An outline of additional anatomical structures that can be seen in a PA chest radiograph. The anterior portions of the ribs are labeled in black and the posterior portions are labeled in white.

28

Figure 1-25 is a lateral radiograph of the same person seen in *Figures 1-23 and 1-24*. Again, as much of the normal anatomy as possible should be considered when viewing the lateral chest radiograph.

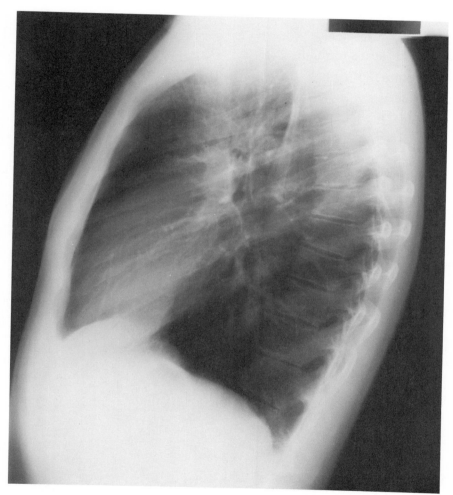

Figure 1-25. An example of a standard lateral chest radiograph.

Figure 1-26 shows the anatomical structures included in a standard lateral chest radiograph (previously shown in Fig. 1-7), as follows:

A—the manubrium

B—the sternum

C—the cardiac silhouette

D—the aortic arch, ascending and descending

E—the trachea, slanting posteriorly in the chest

F—the left bronchus, on end

G—the scapulae

H—the retrosternal air space in the lung

I—the vertebral bodies

R—the right diaphragmatic dome

L—the left diaphragmatic dome

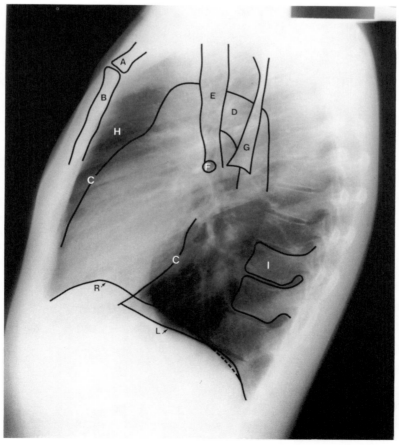

Figure 1-26. An outline of anatomic structures that may be seen on a lateral chest radiograph.

Lobar Anatomy

The division of the lungs into lobes creates **fissures,** which are actually invaginations of the visceral pleura into the interlobar spaces. These fissures are not always seen in chest radiographs.

In the right lung, the fissure separating the right upper lobe (RUL) from the right middle lobe (RML) is called the **minor** or **horizontal fissure;** the separation of the RUL and the RML from the right lower lobe (RLL) is termed the **major fissure** or **oblique fissure.** In the left lung, usually only the major (oblique) fissure separates the left upper lobe (LUL) from the left lower lobe (LLL). The anatomy of the lobar fissures can be seen clearly in *Figure 1-27.*

The relative positioning of the lobes in both frontal and lateral radiographs should be studied thoroughly. Although fissures are not always visible in standard chest radiographs, the viewer should have an idea of approximately where the various lobes are located. In the cases in this text, chest abnormalities will be described relative to specific lobes and, whenever possible, to lobar segments.

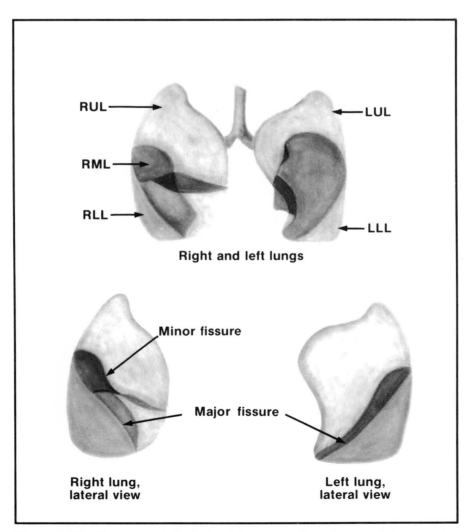

Right and left lungs

Minor fissure

Major fissure

**Right lung,
lateral view**

**Left lung,
lateral view**

Figure 1-27. The anatomical relationships among the pulmonary lobes, creating the lobar fissures.

As exemplified in *Figure 1-28*, the major fissure presents a thin, uniform density to striking x-rays and, therefore, it is not seen on PA chest radiographs. However, if the minor fissure is parallel or head-on to the x-ray beam, sufficient density is created to cause a narrow horizontal line on a radiograph.

Occasionally, the minor fissure is seen in the right lung in a PA radiograph, as seen in *Figure 1-29*. The patient in this figure has a RML pneumonia and the minor fissure is just barely visible, as indicated by the arrow. The same applies to the lateral position, where the x-ray beam may strike parallel to the major (oblique) fissure and cause it to appear in the radiograph *(Fig. 1-30)*.

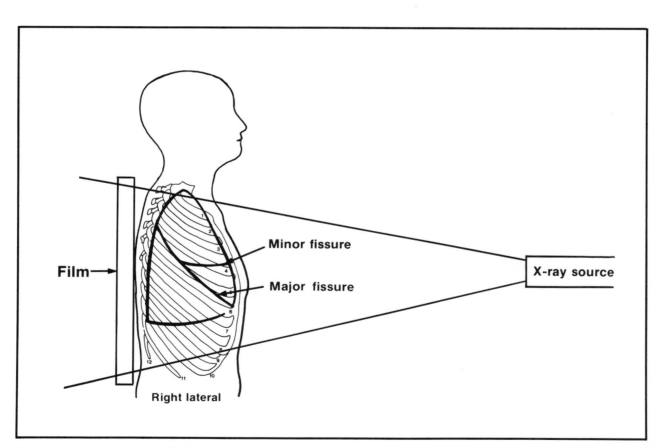

Figure 1-28. The minor fissure (right lung) and the major oblique fissures (right and left lungs) in relation to a striking x-ray beam with AP projection.

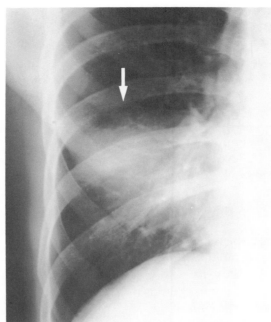

Figure 1-29. The appearance of the minor fissure in the right lung in a patient with pneumonia.

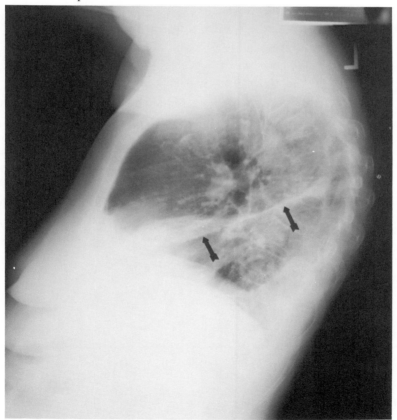

Figure 1-30. The appearance of the major oblique fissure in a lateral radiograph.

METHOD OF INSPECTING THE CHEST RADIOGRAPH

The Technical Quality

Logically, the first step in examining a chest radiograph is to quickly evaluate its quality. The following points should be reviewed before trying to interpret a chest radiograph. First, was the patient's position correct? That is, is the patient straight, and not rotated or slumping? A good clue in evaluating position is to check the relationship of the proximal clavicles to the vertebral column. If the subject is positioned correctly for a PA radiograph, the thoracic vertebral column should exactly bisect a line drawn between the ends of the proximal clavicles, and the sternoclavicular joints and the costophrenic angles should be equidistant from the spine. Otherwise, the relative positions of the hilar shadows cannot be used diagnostically, as discussed earlier.

Second, the exposure quality can be evaluated by determining whether the spinous processes of the vertebrae are visible to the fifth or sixth thoracic level (T5-T6). Usually, such visibility indicates a normal degree of exposure. Many radiology departments, however, are changing to high kilovolt techniques for PA radiographs, in which vertebrae can be seen all the way down the cardiac shadow.

The relative densities seen in the chest form the basis for determining the degree of exposure. For example, the heart is denser than air-filled lungs, thus it is whiter than the lung fields in a normal radiograph. The normal relative density of heart to lung fields becomes evident with continued practice in viewing both normal and abnormal radiographs. Likewise, the heart becomes more radiolucent, or darker, and the lungs become proportionately darker with greater exposure of the radiograph. An overexposed radiograph is referred to as "heavily penetrated." In an overexposed radiograph, the air-filled lung periphery becomes even more radiolucent and gives the appearance of lacking tissue, as in pulmonary emphysema. A clinical term that is often used with very dark lung fields is "burned-out." The problem is to decide whether the dark appearance in the radiograph is caused by overexposure or lack of lung tissue. Evaluate the relative darkness of the different organs. With overexposure, the dark lung fields are seen with a darker than normal, more radiolucent cardiac shadow. With tissue loss, a normally radiolucent cardiac shadow is seen, but very dark, more radiolucent lung fields are evident. Conversely, underexposed lungs may appear to be denser and whiter, as if with infiltrates, but the cardiac shadow is whiter still, with little or no visibility of the thoracic vertebrae.

The third point to review before trying to interpret a chest radiograph involves the extent of inspiration. Was the patient inspiring adequately? The diaphragmatic dome should be at the level of the ninth to eleventh ribs posteriorly. On expiration the lungs have less air, appear cloudier or denser, the diaphragm is raised, and the heart appears to be wider and enlarged. The resulting image is similar to that seen with congestive heart failure. *ON (E) as opposed to (I)*

34

Anatomical Inspection

Once the technical quality of the radiograph has been determined, the next step is to review the entire chest radiograph (both PA and lateral, if available). *Figure 1-31* illustrates an "inside out" approach to looking at chest radiographs, that is, beginning with the mediastinum and proceeding outward to the skin and soft tissue. Some practitioners, however, may prefer the reverse. The point to be emphasized is the need for a *systematic method:* systematically reviewing the film reduces the likelihood of missing important features, especially when distracted by an obvious and striking abnormality. Such a method should become a habit for anyone who frequently views chest radiographs.

Universal advice to those viewing chest radiographs is to describe rather than diagnose what is seen. A chest radiograph alone is not diagnostic; it is only one piece of descriptive information. It is often advantageous to examine the chest radiograph with an open mind, without being biased by any prior clinical knowledge of the patient. This precaution reduces the temptation to see what may not actually be on the radiograph. In concrete terms, this means that only descriptive words, such as shadows, density or patchiness, should be used to discuss the radiograph. One would not say, "I see a bronchopneumonia in the left lower lobe," but instead, "I see a patchy infiltrate," or "I see a streaky density in the left lower lobe." Of course, in actual practice, the radiologist or attending physician knows the patient's clinical history and the other laboratory information, and often has a clinical diagnosis already in mind when looking at the radiograph. Consequently, a density is often seen as "the suggestion of a pneumonia," or it may be correlated with possible causes

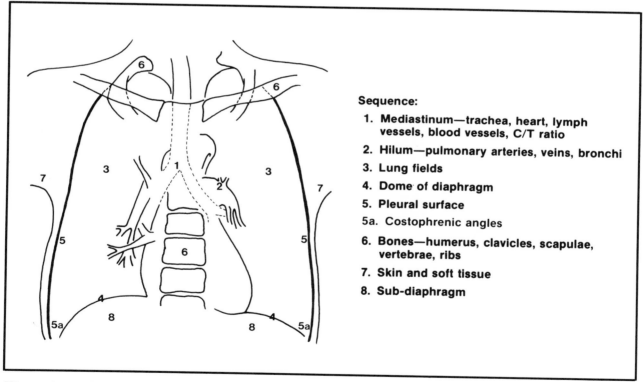

Sequence:

1. **Mediastinum—trachea, heart, lymph vessels, blood vessels, C/T ratio**
2. **Hilum—pulmonary arteries, veins, bronchi**
3. **Lung fields**
4. **Dome of diaphragm**
5. **Pleural surface**
5a. **Costophrenic angles**
6. **Bones—humerus, clavicles, scapulae, vertebrae, ribs**
7. **Skin and soft tissue**
8. **Sub-diaphragm**

Figure 1-31. Sequential inspection of the major areas seen in a chest radiograph using an inside out approach.

of such an appearance without specifying a particular cause. Specifying a cause would amount to a diagnosis from the radiograph itself. Always keep in mind that shadows (on radiographs, as well as on movie screens) can have different causes. For example, a round density in the middle of a lung field in a PA radiograph may be caused by a nipple, or by a tumor.

Review all of the visible anatomy of the mediastinum (*Fig. 1-32*), looking for the trachea, carina, cardiac outline, aortic arch, blood vessels such as the superior vena cava, and the presence of enlarged lymph nodes. Note the cardiothoracic ratio, taking into account the patient's position (PA, AP).

Inspect the hilar region on both sides. Is the left hilum higher than the right, as is usually the case? (*See Figure 1-33.*) Is there an increased density of these vessels, indicating possible engorgement caused by increased pulmonary vascular resistance or other causes? Are enlarged and/or calcified lymph nodes present, as in histoplasmosis, tuberculosis or other infections?

Inspect both lung fields in their entirety out to the periphery (*Fig. 1-34*). Normally, there are visible markings scattered throughout the lungs. The absence of tissue markings might indicate a pneumothorax or the removal of a lung, as immediately after a pneumonectomy. Excess markings may mean fibrosis, compression of lung tissue, interstitial or alveolar edema, or other lesions. Compare the lung fields for symmetry.

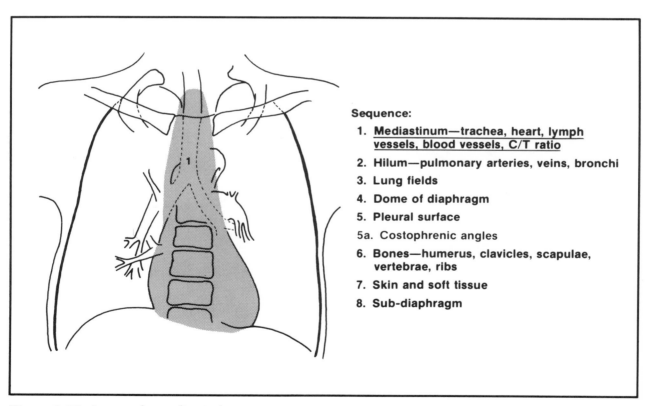

Sequence:

1. **Mediastinum—trachea, heart, lymph vessels, blood vessels, C/T ratio**
2. Hilum—pulmonary arteries, veins, bronchi
3. Lung fields
4. Dome of diaphragm
5. Pleural surface
5a. Costophrenic angles
6. Bones—humerus, clavicles, scapulae, vertebrae, ribs
7. Skin and soft tissue
8. Sub-diaphragm

Figure 1-32. Inspect the mediastinal area.

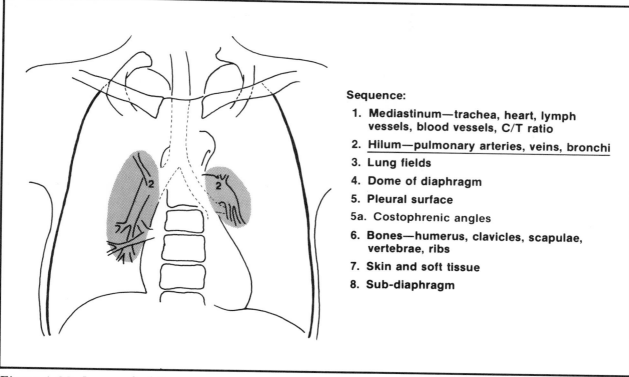

Sequence:

1. **Mediastinum—trachea, heart, lymph vessels, blood vessels, C/T ratio**
2. <u>**Hilum—pulmonary arteries, veins, bronchi**</u>
3. **Lung fields**
4. **Dome of diaphragm**
5. **Pleural surface**
5a. **Costophrenic angles**
6. **Bones—humerus, clavicles, scapulae, vertebrae, ribs**
7. **Skin and soft tissue**
8. **Sub-diaphragm**

Figure 1-33. Inspect the hilar area.

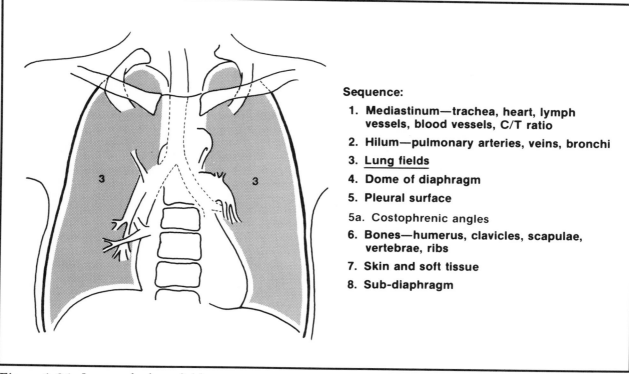

Sequence:

1. **Mediastinum—trachea, heart, lymph vessels, blood vessels, C/T ratio**
2. **Hilum—pulmonary arteries, veins, bronchi**
3. <u>**Lung fields**</u>
4. **Dome of diaphragm**
5. **Pleural surface**
5a. **Costophrenic angles**
6. **Bones—humerus, clavicles, scapulae, vertebrae, ribs**
7. **Skin and soft tissue**
8. **Sub-diaphragm**

Figure 1-34. Inspect the lung fields.

The dome of the diaphragm *(Fig. 1-35)* gives valuable information, such as the level of the diaphragm, or flattening or interdigitation (peaking) above the diaphragm (seen with chronic obstructive disease), or unequal excursion (seen with unilateral diaphragmatic paralysis). The left dome is normally slightly lower than the right due to elevation by the liver, located under the right hemidiaphragm.

Follow the pleural surface (edges of the lung) around the entire perimeter of the lung fields. Note the sharpness of the costophrenic angles, which reveals whether they are free from effusion *(Fig. 1-36)*. Normally, the intrapleural space is not visible unless it is occupied by a mass, air (pneumothorax), or fluid (pleural effusion).

The bony structure of the chest should be clearly visible in a radiograph. Each bone should be examined along its entire length *(Fig. 1-37)*. Examine the humerus, clavicles, scapulae, ribs and vertebrae in the figure. Are the intercostal spacings symmetrical and even? Have any ribs been fractured, or do any ribs display notching? Occasionally, in the absence of a known trauma, a hole may be seen in a rib.

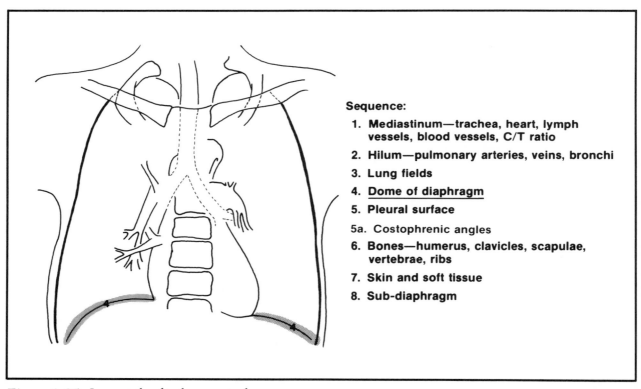

Sequence:

1. **Mediastinum—trachea, heart, lymph vessels, blood vessels, C/T ratio**
2. **Hilum—pulmonary arteries, veins, bronchi**
3. **Lung fields**
4. **Dome of diaphragm**
5. **Pleural surface**
5a. **Costophrenic angles**
6. **Bones—humerus, clavicles, scapulae, vertebrae, ribs**
7. **Skin and soft tissue**
8. **Sub-diaphragm**

Figure 1-35. Inspect the diaphragmatic domes.

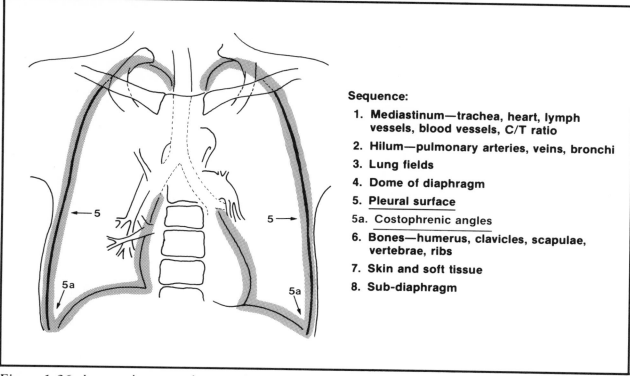

Sequence:

1. **Mediastinum—trachea, heart, lymph vessels, blood vessels, C/T ratio**
2. **Hilum—pulmonary arteries, veins, bronchi**
3. **Lung fields**
4. **Dome of diaphragm**
5. <u>**Pleural surface**</u>
5a. Costophrenic angles
6. **Bones—humerus, clavicles, scapulae, vertebrae, ribs**
7. **Skin and soft tissue**
8. **Sub-diaphragm**

Figure 1-36. Inspect the circumference of the lungs to evaluate the pleural surface and costophrenic angles.

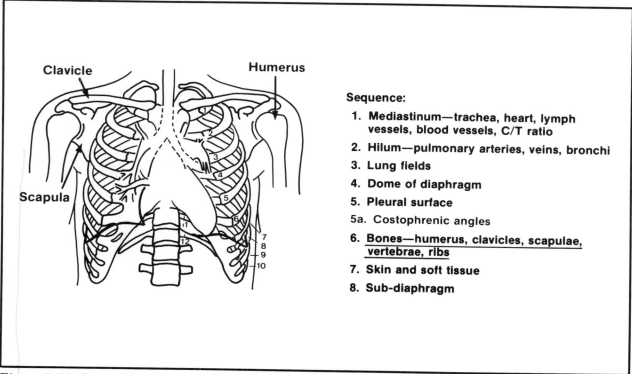

Sequence:

1. **Mediastinum—trachea, heart, lymph vessels, blood vessels, C/T ratio**
2. **Hilum—pulmonary arteries, veins, bronchi**
3. **Lung fields**
4. **Dome of diaphragm**
5. **Pleural surface**
5a. Costophrenic angles
6. <u>**Bones—humerus, clavicles, scapulae, vertebrae, ribs**</u>
7. **Skin and soft tissue**
8. **Sub-diaphragm**

Figure 1-37. Inspect the appearance of bony structures in the thorax.

Continuing outward from the mediastinum, inspect the soft tissue (*Fig. 1-38*). Are any breast shadows evident? Do any densities appear in the soft tissue or the axillary regions? Subcutaneous air bubbles give a distinctive appearance as lucencies and may often be seen after a tracheostomy or a pneumothorax.

Finally, consider the visible area below the diaphragm (*Fig. 1-39*). Is there a dark line indicating free air under the diaphragm, which may occur following abdominal surgery (e.g., a cholecystectomy) or peritoneal abscess? Often, the stomach bubble appears under the left hemidiaphragm with an air-fluid line, which helps determine the patient's position at the time the radiograph was taken.

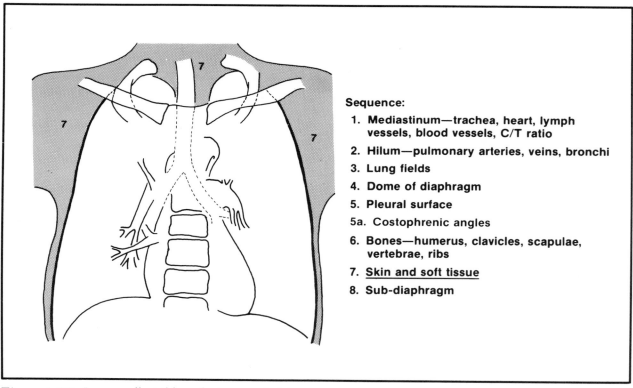

Sequence:

1. **Mediastinum—trachea, heart, lymph vessels, blood vessels, C/T ratio**

2. **Hilum—pulmonary arteries, veins, bronchi**

3. **Lung fields**

4. **Dome of diaphragm**

5. **Pleural surface**

5a. **Costophrenic angles**

6. **Bones—humerus, clavicles, scapulae, vertebrae, ribs**

7. **Skin and soft tissue**

8. **Sub-diaphragm**

Figure 1-38. Inspect all visible soft tissue and skin.

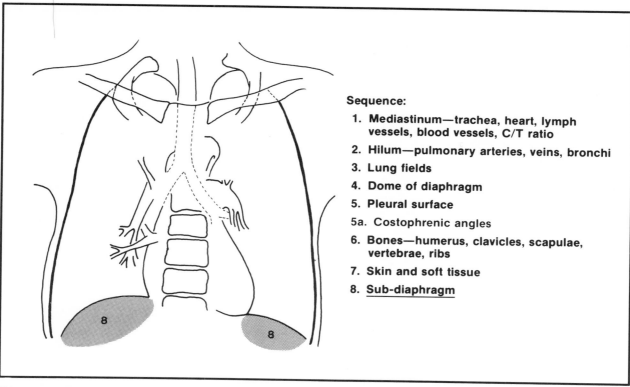

Sequence:

1. **Mediastinum—trachea, heart, lymph vessels, blood vessels, C/T ratio**
2. **Hilum—pulmonary arteries, veins, bronchi**
3. **Lung fields**
4. **Dome of diaphragm**
5. **Pleural surface**
5a. **Costophrenic angles**
6. **Bones—humerus, clavicles, scapulae, vertebrae, ribs**
7. **Skin and soft tissue**
8. **Sub-diaphragm**

Figure 1-39. Inspect the region visible below the diaphragm.

Pleural and Extrapleural Lesions

The pleura is a double-walled, membranous sac enclosing each lung. The wall closest to the lung is the visceral pleura. The outside wall is the parietal pleura. The intrapleural space is potential and not directly visible in a chest radiograph. There are two types of abnormalities involving the pleurae that can be differentiated in chest radiographs: extrapleural lesions, which are abnormalities outside both visceral and parietal pleurae, and those between the two pleural surfaces, such as pleural effusion, pneumothorax or hemothorax (Fig. 1-40).

Extrapleural lesions can be differentiated from pleural effusions primarily by the difference in the border of the density. As seen in *Figure 1-41*, an extrapleural lesion lies outside both visceral and parietal pleurae, compressing pleurae and lung tissue into a sharper, better-defined border.

By contrast, a pleural effusion presents a hazy, indistinct border, simply shading off to a less dense appearance. The pleural effusion lies in the intrapleural space, cupping around the lung tissue to produce the characteristic diffuseness seen in *Figure 1-42*. If the patient is supine when an AP radiograph is taken, fluid may spread out thinly in the pleural space around the back of the lung. Upright, the costophrenic angle is obliterated because the denser collection of fluid gravitates to the base of the pleural space.

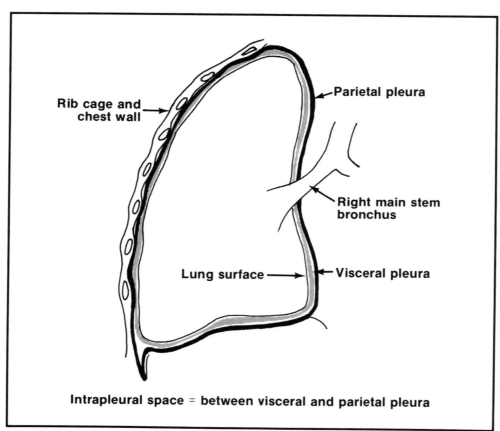

Rib cage and chest wall

Parietal pleura

Right main stem bronchus

Lung surface

Visceral pleura

Intrapleural space = between visceral and parietal pleura

Figure 1-40. The basic anatomy of the chest wall, pleural surfaces, and lung.

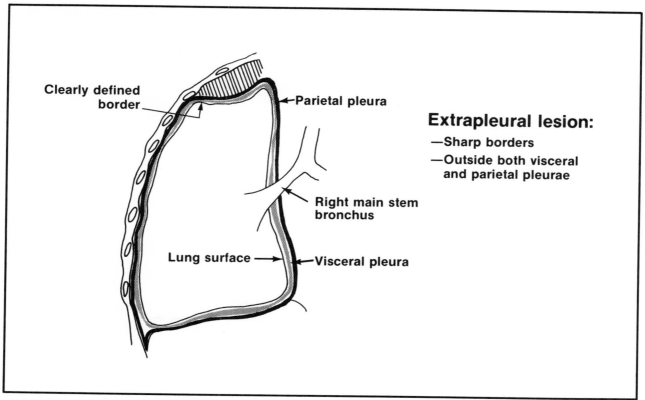

Figure 1-41. Description of an extrapleural density or lesion.

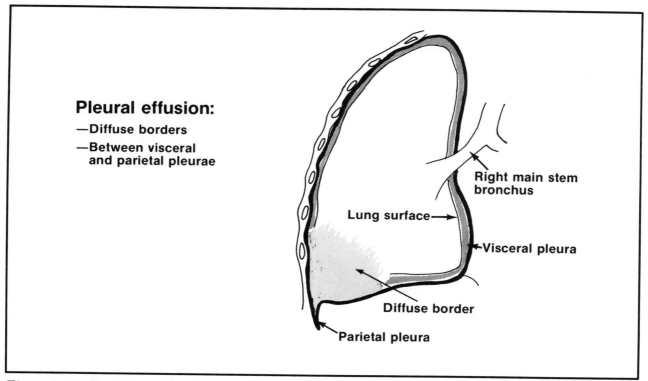

Figure 1-42. Description of a pleural effusion.

The classic appearance of an extrapleural density is presented in *Figure 1-43*, an AP supine chest radiograph of a young female following a gunshot wound. The figure shows that the patient is slightly rotated to the right and that the radiograph is extremely overpenetrated. On inspecting the lung fields, it is immediately apparent that the right lung field is much denser than the left. This density is caused by fluid (blood) spreading out in the posterior pleural space. Also, the right costophrenic angle has been obliterated by this same fluid. Following the right pleural border, the obvious density of one of the bullets is seen near the seventh rib posteriorly. Observe the sharply demarcated density projecting in from the right thoracic wall. The arrowheads point out the border. This is a typical sign of an extrapleural density, which, in this case, is blood. The blood is outside of the parietal pleura. Note also the posteriorly fractured ninth rib near the edge of the right chest (circle), as well as a second bullet lying near the twelfth thoracic vertebra (T-12), indicated by an arrow. A nasogastric tube is also seen in place.

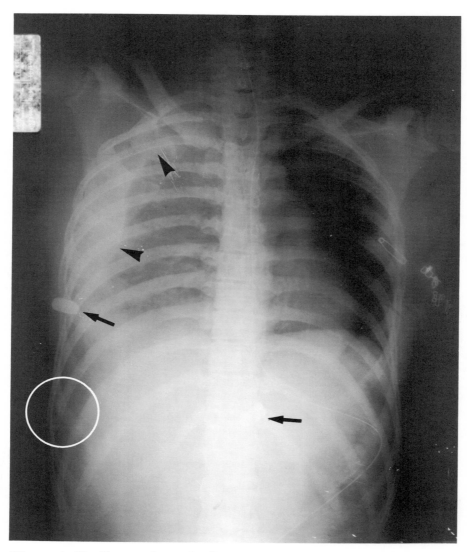

Figure 1-43. Chest radiograph illustrating an extrapleural density (arrowheads). Note the bullets near the seventh rib posteriorly and the twelfth thoracic vertebra (arrows), and the posteriorly fractured ninth rib (circle).

The Silhouette Sign

The silhouette sign is a chest radiologic finding that is often helpful in localizing a density or shadow.

The principle of the silhouette sign is as follows:

A mass or consolidation touching a border of the heart, aorta or diaphragm will obliterate that border on the radiograph. A mass or consolidation that is not in physical contact with the border of such an organ or vessel will not obliterate that border, even though mass and organ are superimposed on the particular radiograph.

The obliteration of a border's delineation by a mass is evidence of the **silhouette sign,** indicating physical contiguity of mass and border and, therefore, loss of border visibility.

In *Figure 1-44*, a model of the heart and aorta is sketched, both from a superior view and an anterior view. In **A**, with sufficient x-ray penetration, the line of the aorta would be visible through the cardiac shadow because the aorta and heart are not physically in contact, even though they are superimposed in the frontal projection. In **B**, the heart model is in a box of fluid. Because the fluid is in physical contact with the border of the heart, the border disappears, giving the frontal appearance shown in **B**; however, the aorta's edges can still be seen because they are separated from the heart and fluid. Finally, in **C**, the border of the aorta disappears once it reaches the box of fluid, although the cardiac outline remains visible despite superimposition of the box of fluid. Felson (1973) reproduces actual radiographs of such a model.

If only the frontal projections were available (for example, a PA radiograph) of the situations in

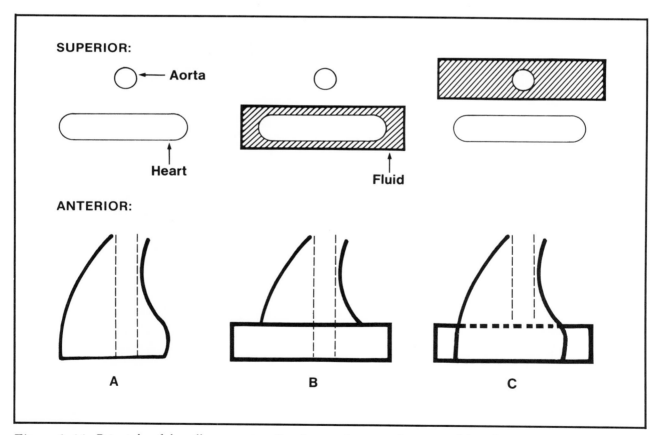

Figure 1-44. Principle of the silhouette sign. See the text for an explanation of this phenomenon. *Adapted from: Chest Roentgenology. Philadelphia, W.B. Saunders Co., 1973.*

B and C, the depth, or three-dimensional location, of the fluid could be obtained. The silhouette sign in **B** involves loss of the heart border; therefore, the fluid is touching the heart, indicating a more anterior location. The silhouette sign in **C** involves the aorta; therefore, the fluid surrounds the aorta, indicating a more posterior location.

In the right lung, the middle lobe is next to the right border of the heart. Therefore, consolidation of the right middle lobe, which occurs in pneumonia, results in loss of the right heart border. This fact can aid in distinguishing right middle lobe involvement from posterior densities of the lower lobe, which is not in contact with the right heart border.

In the left lung, infiltrates or consolidation of the lingula (lower division of the left upper lobe) obscure the left cardiac border.

Silhouette sign of the right and left heart borders aids in localizing infiltrates or consolidation to the right middle lobe and to the lingular region of the left lung.

The silhouette sign cannot be seen in the radiograph shown in *Figure 1-45*. The descending aorta, marked by an arrow, can be seen through the cardiac shadow, indicating that the heart and aorta are not in physical contact. If they were, a uniform shadow would be seen in the radiograph, and the aorta would simply disappear into the heart shadow.

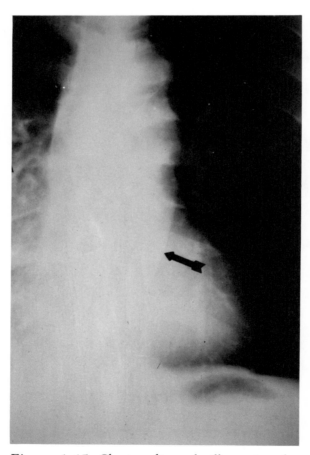

Figure 1-45. Chest radiograph illustrating the absence of the silhouette sign, showing the superimposed, but physically distinct heart and descending aorta.

46

The Air Bronchogram

The air bronchogram is another radiologic sign that may be seen with some forms of pulmonary consolidation, particularly parenchymal consolidation. Normally, in the expanded, air-filled lung, the bronchi and bronchioles are not visible. The bronchi are, of course, buried in surrounding alveoli, and both bronchi and alveoli are air-filled. Because there is no difference in density, the airways are not visible in the chest radiograph. The walls of the airways are not dense enough to create a shadow. However, if the surrounding alveolar tissue becomes consolidated while the bronchi remain clear, the bronchi can be seen radiographically, and an air bronchogram results. The airways are then less dense and appear darker (more radiolucent), outlined by the denser surrounding parenchyma, which is lighter.

Figures 1-46 and 1-47 are AP and lateral chest radiographs illustrating an air bronchogram seen with respiratory distress syndrome in a neonate. A large bubble of abdominal gas, which is normal, can be seen below the left hemidiaphragm. Both lung fields are increased in density and have a granular appearance. A symmetrical pattern of radiating air bronchograms is visible in both the AP and lateral radiographs. In the AP radiograph (*Fig. 1-46*), the bronchogram can be seen over the area of the heart, and particularly over the left lung, as fine, branching dark shadows (circle). Arrows indicate another air bronchogram. The lateral radiograph gives an especially striking view of the tracheobronchial branching depicted in the air bronchogram. The presence of the air bronchogram confirms the parenchymal involvement of infant respiratory distress syndrome.

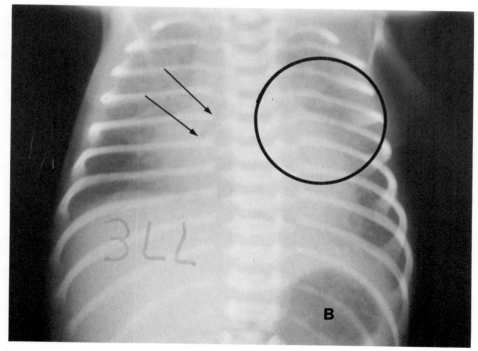

Figure 1-46. AP chest radiograph of a neonate, showing an air bronchogram on the right side (arrows) and several on the left (circle). A bubble (B) of abdominal gas is clearly visible.

Diagnostically, the appearance of an air bronchogram within a density on the radiograph indicates an alveolar consolidation because this condition is required to produce such an image. However, if a density is seen on the radiograph without the presence of an air bronchogram, nothing can be concluded regarding the density's location. Such a density, or lesion, without the presence of an air bronchogram could be extrapulmonary (pleural or mediastinal) or intrapulmonary with airless bronchi. A density in the absence of an air bronchogram is, therefore, an ambiguous finding that precludes parenchymal or nonparenchymal localization.

The technical quality of a chest radiograph, especially the degree of exposure, can affect the appearance of an air bronchogram. Generally, an air bronchogram is very faint and difficult to see. Underexposed radiographs may mask the presence of an air bronchogram. Finally, if there is doubt regarding whether a shadow represents bronchi within consolidated alveoli, branching of the radiolucent lines confirms that the airways are being seen.

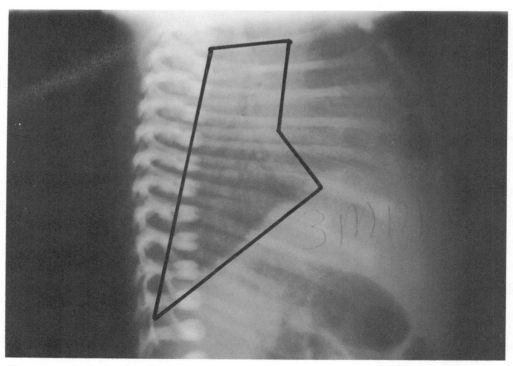

Figure 1-47. Lateral radiograph of a neonate, with an air bronchogram outlining much of the tracheobronchial branching.

RADIONUCLIDE PERFUSION AND VENTILATION SCANS

A discussion of the nuclear medicine techniques in radiology is far beyond the scope and intent of this text. However, lung scans, both perfusion and ventilation, are extremely useful techniques that are common in critical care medicine and are often used in conjunction with the traditional chest radiograph. In Part Two of this text, both perfusion and ventilation lung scans will be seen in several of the cases presented. Hence, a brief description of both types of scans follows. The intent of this discussion on perfusion and ventilation scanning is only to give the practitioner a basic familiarity with what is represented by a scan. The reader desiring more detail on the use of perfusion and ventilation scans in obstructive lung disease and pulmonary embolism is referred to Taplin and Chopra (1978) and Secker-Walker and Siegel (1973).

Perfusion Scan

To obtain an image of pulmonary perfusion, such as the one seen in *Figure 1-48*, a radioactive tracer material is injected intravenously. The tracer material is sized to become trapped in the pulmonary circulation, where it will provide an image of the distribution of pulmonary blood flow for a suitable scanning camera.

The usual procedure is to inject small clumps of albumin, called macroaggregates, tagged with a radioactive material such as iodine 131 or technetium 99m. Pulmonary capillaries are approximately 8 to 10μ in diameter; therefore, radioactive particles of 20 to 50μ lodge in the blood vessels. The particles eventually break down, pass through the pulmonary circulation and are removed by the liver and spleen. Because the number of capillaries far exceeds the number of particles injected, no significant effect on pulmonary hemodynamics results from this procedure.

Following injection of the particles, the lung fields are scanned for radioactivity, usually from the anterior, posterior and lateral surfaces. The scan gives a picture of lung perfusion, with the dark areas representing a good concentration of radioactivity and, therefore, a good blood flow. Light areas and areas with decreased density on the scan are interpreted as having absent or decreased blood flow. Currently, perfusion scans can be performed relatively quickly and with minimal radiation exposure.

The perfusion scan shown in *Figure 1-48* is a posterior scan. The right lung is on the viewer's left. The asymmetrical appearance of the right and left lungs is obvious, indicating severely decreased blood flow in the right lung, which appears much lighter on the scan. This case is discussed in more detail in Part Two in the section entitled "Pulmonary Embolism and Perfusion Scan." Some general principles concerning the clinical application of perfusion scans in the diagnosis of pulmonary embolism are offered there.

Unfortunately, perfusion scan defects are not specific to any one cause. Any of the following can cause diminished regional blood flow: pulmonary emboli, loss of the vascular bed in chronic lung disease, lung abscess, compression of lung by masses, bullae, atelectasis or consolidating pneumonia. Cowan (1978) gives a useful summary of the perfusion scan technique and its clinical applications.

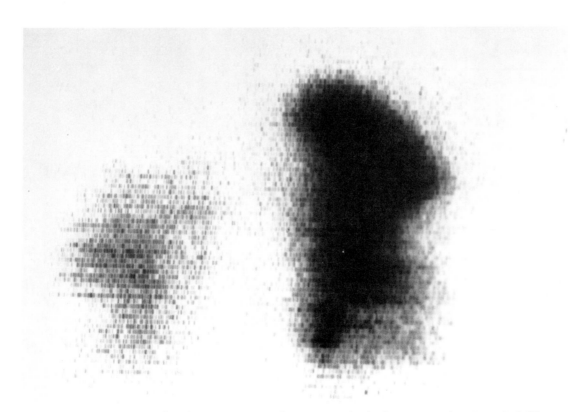

Figure 1-48. An example of a posterior perfusion scan (right lung is on the viewer's left).

50

Ventilation Scan

There are two nuclear medicine techniques for assessing ventilation: radioaerosol inhalation and radioactive gas inhalation, with subsequent camera scanning as in the perfusion technique. The radioaerosol technique is less common and employs a nebulized solution with a radioactive tag. The aerosol can be administered via a positive-pressure breathing device with a micronebulizer or by means of an ultrasonic nebulizer. All of the considerations of particle size, penetration and deposition that are familiar to those persons involved in aerosol therapies are applicable to the radioaerosol technique. For example, the aerosol particle size must be less than 2μ to reach the lung periphery.

The more common technique for ventilation scanning uses radioactive gases, such as xenon 133. The patient is connected to a rebreathing circuit, and a bolus of labeled gas is introduced into the circuit as the patient inhales. The patient then holds his or her breath while an image is made of the initial single-breath distribution of the labeled gas. Further images are made during rebreathing, representing an equilibration phase. At the conclusion of the procedure, the patient is switched to room air, and images are made of the wash-out phase as the expired radioactive gas is collected to prevent room contamination. A normal ventilation study would show approximately uniform lung distribution of the gas during the initial inspiration and breath-hold, little change throughout the equilibration phase, and rapid wash-out.

A ventilation scan using xenon 133 and the gas inhalation technique is presented in *Figure 1-49*. Details of the clinical case and its radiographic interpretation are given in Part Two (see section entitled "Right Upper Lobe Bulla"). *Figure 1-49* is a ventilation scan from the equilibration phase; the right lung is on the viewer's left. As with a perfusion image, dark areas reflect the presence of the radioactive substance and, hence, regional ventilation. An area of lighter density or no activity (no darkness) represents a lack of ventilation. There are a number of possible causes of abnormal ventilation, such as: airway occlusion from mucus or a foreign body, bronchospasm, loss of elasticity (emphysema), alveolar consolidation from pneumonia or pulmonary edema,

and airway compression from a mass. The washout phase is frequently very useful in assessing ventilation and can indicate the air trapping and delayed clearance that are common in obstructive lung disease. In the case seen in *Figure 1-49*, there is a noticeable asymmetry between the right and left apices. The lack of activity in the right apex corresponds to an area of poor ventilation.

In summary, with perfusion and ventilation images obtained using radioactive tracers, the dark areas indicate good perfusion or ventilation, respectively. The basic principle to be remembered is that the degree of activity seen during scanning corresponds to the degree of perfusion or ventilation.

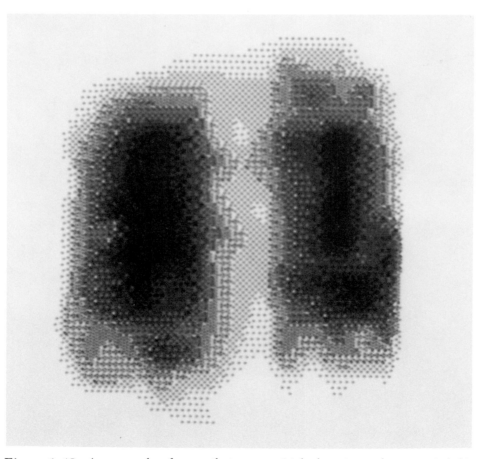

Figure 1-49. An example of a ventilation scan (right lung is on the viewer's left).

Part Two
Selected Abnormalities on Chest Radiographs

Inspecting Chest Radiographs

Part Two presents a series of cases exemplifying the chest abnormalities of special interest to the respiratory and critical care practitioner. The discussion of each case is based on an actual radiograph. Many cases are illustrated by a series of chest radiographs. This can be useful for recognizing progressive changes in appearance for a given condition, such as a pneumothorax before and after insertion of a chest tube.

When reviewing the cases in Part Two, it is important to keep the principles discussed in Part One clearly in mind. In particular, each chest radiograph should be reviewed using the systematic method of inspection discussed in Part One of this text. In Part Two, the application of this method is frequently noted when introducing the chest radiograph for a new case.

Main Stem Bronchial Intubation

One of the most important uses of chest radiographs for practitioners in respiratory and critical care is the visual confirmation of endotracheal tube position. This is especially true in intensive care units or whenever prolonged intubation is anticipated. Unless the tube position has been verified by bronchoscopy, it is essential that the placement be checked using a chest radiograph; bilateral breath-sound equality is not sufficient to verify proper positioning, especially if continued mechanical ventilation is to be employed. The patient seen in *Figure 2-1* is a 43-year-old female who, because of progressive respiratory failure, was intubated by an anesthesiologist at 2:00 p.m. and was placed on a ventilator. *Figure 2-1* is a chest radiograph taken 20 minutes after intubation.

The viewer may assume that the radiograph is an AP radiograph because the scapulae are visible in the lung fields and the heart appears magnified. In fact, this is the case. The viewer should note that the radiograph is slightly underexposed since the vertebrae are not visible through the cardiac shadow. Of prime importance in this radiograph is the position of the endotracheal tube. The arrow in the center points to the main carina, which is somewhat difficult to see. The arrow to the viewer's left points to the tip of the endotracheal tube, obviously well into the right main stem bronchus. However, at the time of intubation, breath sounds were thought to be equal bilaterally. In this case, the anesthesiologist who performed the intubation was called to an emergency and did not view the radiograph. The ICU staff assumed that the radiograph had been checked and that the tube was in good position.

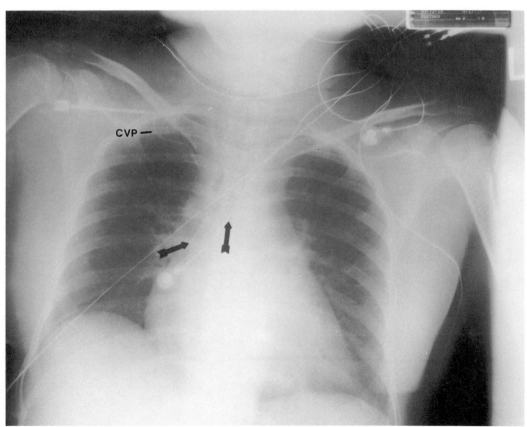

Figure 2-1. Chest radiograph showing endotracheal tube placement in right main stem bronchus (arrow on the viewer's left). The arrow in the center points to the main carina. Also, note the central venous pressure line (CVP) and the cardiac monitor electrodes and wires.

A central venous pressure (CVP) line, which enters from the patient's right subclavian vein, and several cardiac monitor electrodes with wires can be seen in *Figure 2-1*. The cardiothoracic (C-T) ratio is somewhat enlarged, and, because this patient has a history of congestive heart failure (CHF), it is difficult to determine whether this increased C-T ratio was caused by left ventricular hypertrophy, or the magnification that is normally seen in an AP radiograph, or both.

Figure 2-2 is a close-up of the carina and endotracheal tube of the same patient. Once again the endotracheal tube is clearly well into the main stem bronchus. The radiopaque line marking the endotracheal tube is better seen in this close-up view.

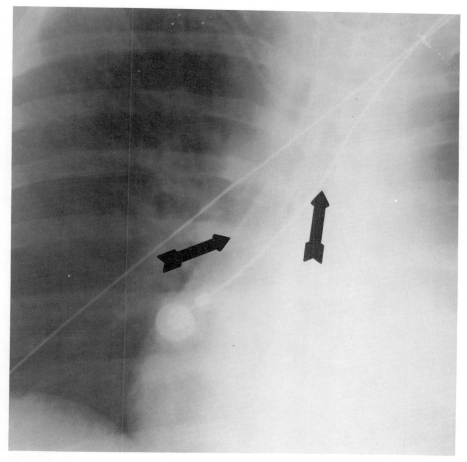

Figure 2-2. Close-up of the carina and endotracheal tube.

At 4:00 p.m. on the same day, the patient had a cardiac arrest. Following successful resuscitation, breath sounds were absent over the left chest. Another AP chest radiograph was obtained at 4:30 p.m. (*Fig. 2-3*). This radiograph is better exposed and shows that the endotracheal tube is still in the right main stem bronchus. Furthermore, there is a striking white-out of the left lung. Such a hemithorax white-out can be caused by a number of factors, including pneumonectomy, pleural effusion, hemothorax and atelectasis. In this case, based on the clinical history and the right main stem intubation, the patient was diagnosed as having complete atelectasis of the left lung.

Figure 2-4 is a close-up of the radiograph shown in *Figure 2-3*, clearly demonstrating that the endotracheal tube remains in the right main stem bronchus. When this radiograph was viewed and the problem was determined, the tube was retracted several centimeters to a level above the carina. The patient was then sighed with a manual resuscitator bag for several minutes, and another chest radiograph was obtained at 5:00 p.m. (*Fig. 2-5*). This is an AP radiograph with good exposure. As indicated by the arrows, the tip of the tube is now about 1 cm above the carina, although it could still be retracted slightly for optimal position (about 2 cm above the main carina). The left lung has reinflated, although there are still areas of atelectasis and infiltrate scattered throughout the left lung field; the left heart border and the diaphragm are partially obscured. The CVP line and EKG monitor leads are still present in this radiograph.

Figure 2-6 is a close-up of the tip of the tube (the arrow on the viewer's left) and the carina (the arrow on the viewer's right).

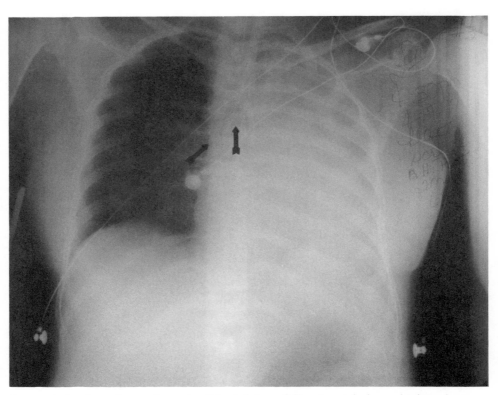

Figure 2-3. Complete atelectasis of the left lung following right bronchial intubation.

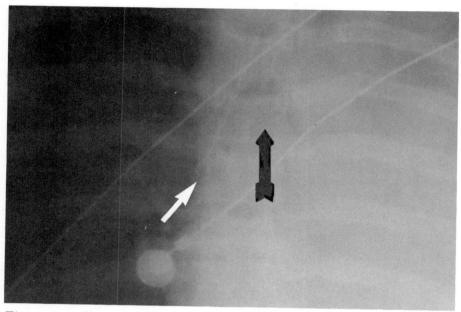

Figure 2-4. Close-up of the endotracheal tube position (arrow on the viewer's left).

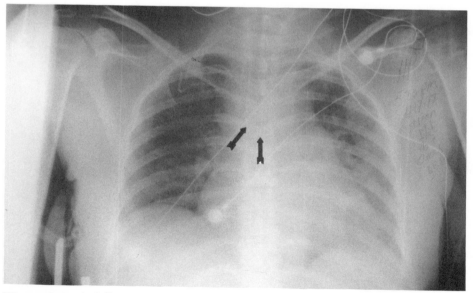

Figure 2-5. A follow-up radiograph showing retraction of the endotracheal tube (arrow on the viewer's left) and reexpansion of the left lung.

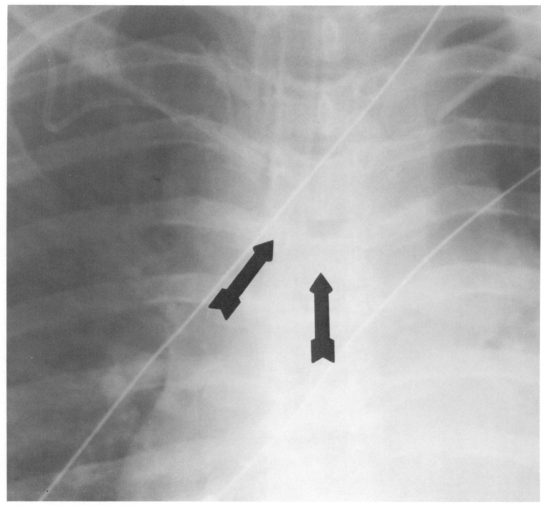

Figure 2-6. Close-up of the endotracheal tube position (arrow on the viewer's left) and carina (arrow in the center).

Tracheostomy Tube

Tracheostomy tubes are a common type of endotracheal tube seen in chest radiographs of patients with some types of chronic pulmonary disease or patients requiring long-term mechanical ventilation. If the tracheostomy tube is metal (e.g., the Jackson silver tube), the outline in the radiograph will be extremely clear; even the plastic tube shown in the AP chest radiograph in *Figure 2-7* gives a definite outline.

To review the radiograph systematically, as suggested in Part One, note that the radiograph is probably an anteroposterior (AP) radiograph, as evidenced by the following: the scapulae have not been rotated out of the lung fields, and the heart shadow is larger, which is consistent with AP magnification. Most decisively, however, check the radiology report or the protective jacket of the radiograph to determine the type of projection.

In *Figure 2-7*, the patient's position is good and there is normal penetration and exposure of the film, as seen in the alignment of clavicles and the visibility of vertebrae. On further examination, a breast mass is evident, indicating that the patient is probably a female.

The tracheostomy tube is being viewed head-on; therefore, the curved portion cannot be seen. The distal tip, inserted inside the trachea, is marked with an arrow. The tracheal shadow is fairly visible, but the carina cannot be seen. *Figure 2-8* better shows the position of this type of tube. This radiograph, a lateral of the same person, gives a dramatic picture of the tracheostomy tube and its insertion into the trachea. The tracheal shadow is clear, with a dark circle below the arrow where the bronchus branches almost directly parallel to the x-ray beam. The same point that was marked

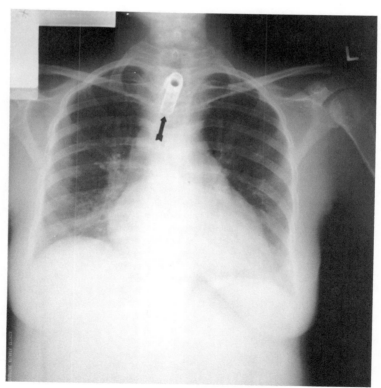

Figure 2-7. Appearance of a tracheostomy tube in an AP chest radiograph (arrow).

with an arrow in the AP radiograph in *Figure 2-7* is similarly marked in this figure.

Subcutaneous emphysema is sometimes visible on radiographs of recently tracheotomized patients. It has the texture of "Rice Krispies" on palpation of the affected tissues, and the air in the tissues appears more radiolucent than the denser skin and soft tissues in the radiograph. The entire skin and soft tissues of the patient's neck and chest should be checked radiographically for air shadows. No evidence of subcutaneous air is present in the patient shown in *Figures 2-7 and 2-8*.

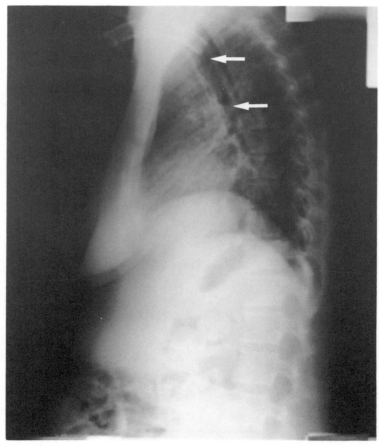

Figure 2-8. Appearance of a tracheostomy tube on a lateral radiograph. The distal tip is marked with an arrow (top). Also, note where the bronchus branches (bottom arrow).

Pneumothorax on Inspiration and Expiration

One of the major concerns of critical care personnel is determining the presence of a pneumothorax, especially in patients with supported ventilation. The case shown in *Figure 2-9* and in succeeding figures provides a good example of the appearance of a pneumothorax. It should help you to recognize the presence of a pneumothorax in less obvious cases. This particular radiograph is a PA projection (scapulae rotated out), the patient is standing up (horizontal air-fluid line in the stomach), the technical quality of the radiograph is good (degree of exposure and positioning), and the patient is probably a female (breast shadows evident). The patient is fully inspired, with the diaphragm at the eleventh rib level posteriorly. A faint vertical density is evident beginning at the fourth rib posteriorly in the left lung field. This density extends in a downward arc, approaching, but not touching, the chest wall. Find and follow this line of density, which is the edge of the pneumothorax, before proceeding. Note that the left costophrenic angle is blunted, as with fluid.

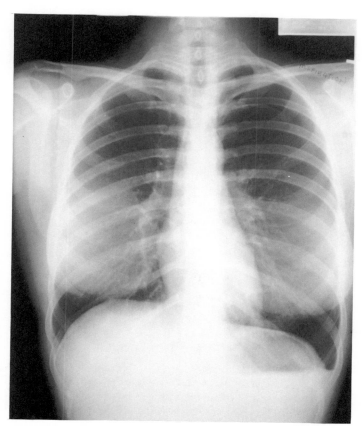

Figure 2-9. Left-sided pneumothorax seen on inspiration. A faint vertical density is evident beginning at the fourth rib posteriorly in the left lung field.

In *Figure 2-10*, the pneumothorax in the left chest is now marked with arrows, outlining its position. The characteristic features to look for when a pneumothorax is suspected is the absence of lung tissue markings and the presence of a border of lung tissue. Observe that the apex of the lung tissue is seen in the fourth intercostal space, and note the difference above and below the lung border. There are absolutely no small tissue markings above the lung, exhibiting an extremely clear appearance in the third intercostal space (right side of *Figure 2-10* in the rectangular area free from obscuring rib shadows). Remember that lungs are air-filled and are not usually dense, but there are normally some markings caused by a small amount of radiation absorption by tissue. In contrast, the pneumothorax is only air; there is nothing in the pleural space, which is now air-filled, to absorb the x-rays. At the same time, the more the lung collapses and is compressed, the denser it will appear in a radiograph, making the diagnosis of pneumothorax more and more obvious. The trachea does not appear to be shifted, and subcutaneous emphysema is not visible. No chest tubes are evident at this point. Compare *Figure 2-10*, in which the patient is inspiring, to *Figure 2-11*, which shows an expiratory phase.

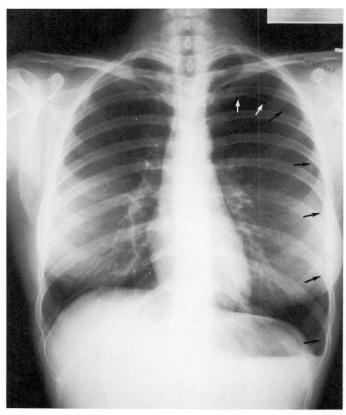

Figure 2-10. Pneumothorax. Arrows indicate the border of the pneumothorax during inspiration. Note the apex of the lung tissue in the fourth intercostal space (upper arrows) and the difference above and below the lung border.

The expiratory phase, shown in *Figure 2-11*, accentuates the pneumothorax because of the loss of negative intrapleural pressure. Consequently, the apical lung border appears at the level of the fifth rib posteriorly, whereas on inspiration it was at the fourth rib. Similarly, the lateral border of the lung is farther inward from the chest wall. Other changes associated with the respiratory phase become apparent when *Figure 2-11* is compared with the preceding inspiratory view. The diaphragm is higher, approaching the tenth rib posteriorly. As a result, the heart appears wider, and the lung bases appear much lighter or denser, with crowded bronchial markings. Part of the lightness (dense appearance) in the bases is caused by a breast shadow, but the difference between inspiration and expiration is still striking. Some radiologists point out that a chest radiograph taken during full expiration can cause changes that simulate congestive heart failure (enlarged cardiac shadow) and the effect of pulmonary infiltrates (clouding of the lung bases). When these effects are seen, it is particularly important to know the level of the diaphragm and the patient's clinical history, if possible.

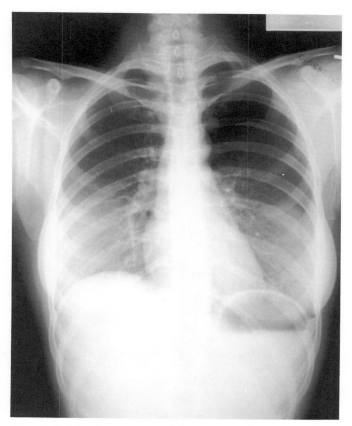

Figure 2-11. Appearance of the pneumothorax on expiration. Compare with Figures 2-9 and 2-10.

The expiratory view of the left pneumothorax is outlined with arrows in *Figure 2-12*, although critical care personnel should be able to find this abnormality without assistance. Often, when a pneumothorax is very small and difficult to detect on an inspiratory radiograph, an expiratory radiograph can accentuate it and provide the practitioner a picture of the lung tissue border not seen on inspiration.

A lateral radiograph of the same patient shows that it is very difficult, and often impossible, to see a pneumothorax on a lateral radiograph *(Fig. 2-13)*. The pneumothorax is evident at one point in the anterior chest. Before proceeding to *Figure 2-14*, where arrows indicate the lung border, look for the edge of the collapsed lung. The two domes of the diaphragm can be seen, and the anterior and posterior diaphragmatic troughs are clear. There

is one other finding in the breast shadow that is not normally seen. Try to locate it before going on.

Both findings on the lateral film are marked with arrows in *Figure 2-14*. Compare your judgment with these results. First, a portion of the collapsed lung border can be seen in the upper anterior portion of the chest, just in front of the aortic arch. Because of the superimposition of right and left lungs and dense shoulder tissue, the rest of the pneumothorax cannot be seen. The second finding (not pathologic) is the presence of breast implants in the shadow created by the breast tissue. The difference in density between normal tissue and the implant is readily apparent in the vertically oriented, concave line indicated by arrows. The remainder of the chest is unremarkable.

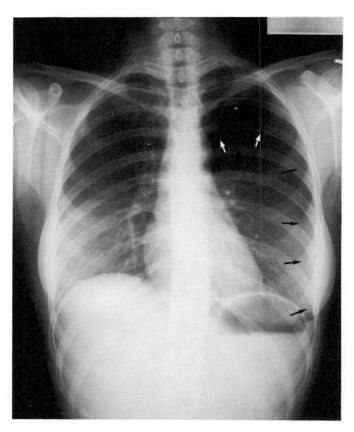

Figure 2-12. Pneumothorax. Arrows indicate the changed pneumothorax border with expiration.

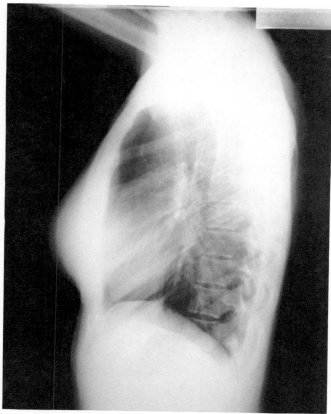

Figure 2-13. Lateral radiograph taken of the same patient in Figures 2-9 through 2-12.

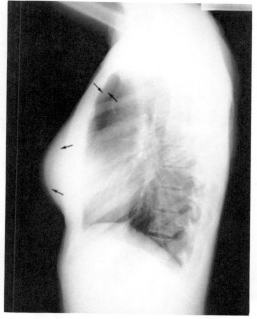

Figure 2-14. Pneumothorax. Arrows outline the lateral view of the pneumothorax, as well as breast implants.

One Hundred Percent (100%) Pneumothorax with Small Chest Tube

A sequence of four figures (*Fig. 2-15 through 2-18*), chest radiographs taken of an 11-year-old female admitted through the emergency room with *status asthmaticus*, illustrates the complication of a pneumothorax that is secondary to asthma. The patient was treated on admission with intravenous aminophylline and steroids, subcutaneous epinephrine, oxygen, and aerosolized isoetharine (Bronkosol) using a compressed air nebulizer. The patient did not appear to obtain any relief from the original therapy. Isoetharine was administered via an intermittent positive pressure breathing (IPPB) machine. The patient seemed markedly improved following the IPPB treatment, which was reflected in her arterial blood gas values. The patient received IPPB treatments with isoetharine throughout the night and continued to improve. At approximately 9:00 a.m., twelve hours after admission, the patient became very dyspneic, and auscultation revealed the virtual absence of breath sounds on the left. The percussion note on that side was thought to be hyperresonant. *Figure 2-15* is a portable chest radiograph obtained at this point. In this radiograph, a one hundred percent pneumothorax is shown on the left (arrow). Subcutaneous air, which has dissected along the tissue planes, is also visible in both cervical regions and along the lateral thoracic wall.

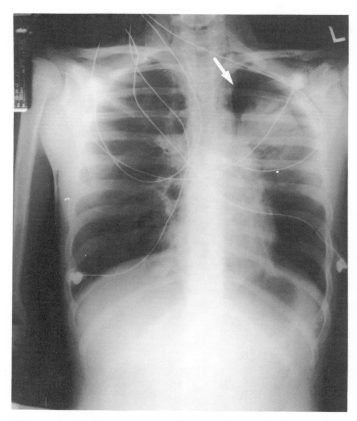

Figure 2-15. Appearance of a 100% left-sided pneumothorax.

A small thoracotomy tube was immediately inserted on the left side, and another portable chest radiograph was obtained (*Fig. 2-16*). The small chest tube is clearly visible as the vertical tubing in the left pleural space, although the lung remains completely collapsed. Arrows indicate the collapsed lung border. Also visible in this radiograph is an increase in the lung markings in the right base.

Because the lung failed to reexpand, the small chest tube was removed and a larger one was inserted. A third chest radiograph was then taken (*Fig. 2-17*). This radiograph is very heavily penetrated, giving both lung fields a very dark appear-ance and making lung markings on both sides difficult to see. However, the larger chest tube, seen entering on the left, almost completely reexpanded the left lung.

Figure 2-18 is a lateral radiograph showing the thoracotomy tube in place. The EKG monitor leads are also visible on the chest wall. Together, *Figures 2-17 and 2-18* give a clear view of the placement of a chest tube for evacuating intrapleural air. The patient in this case continued to improve, the chest tube was removed in three days, and the patient was discharged in good condition one week later.

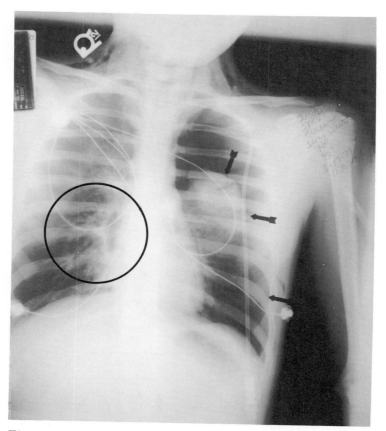

Figure 2-16. Chest radiograph of a pneumothorax following insertion of a small chest tube. Arrows indicate the collapsed lung border. Note the increase in lung markings in the right base (circle).

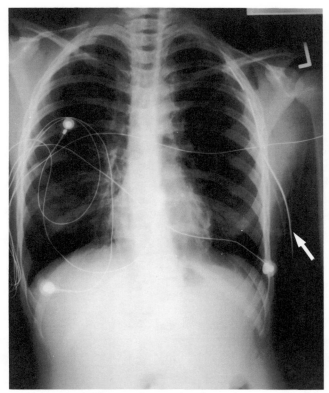

Figure 2-17. Chest radiograph taken after removal of a small chest rube and insertion of a larger tube (arrow), with reexpansion of the left lung.

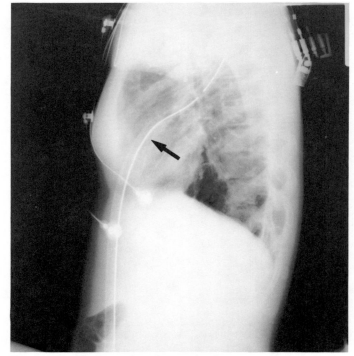

Figure 2-18. Lateral radiograph showing the chest tube (arrow).

Pneumothorax Before and After Chest Tube

The radiograph of a young woman in *Figure 2-19* is somewhat overexposed; but it shows a striking, almost one hundred percent right-sided pneumothorax. The absence of any tissue markings indicates that the intrapleural space is air-filled. Only a portion of the right middle lobe may still be aerated. Note the presence of an air bronchogram outlining several bronchi against the consolidated surrounding lung tissue in the seventh intercostal space, just adjacent to the cardiac shadow. Neither the trachea nor the heart appear shifted. The right costophrenic angle is blunted as with fluid. No subcutaneous emphysema can be seen.

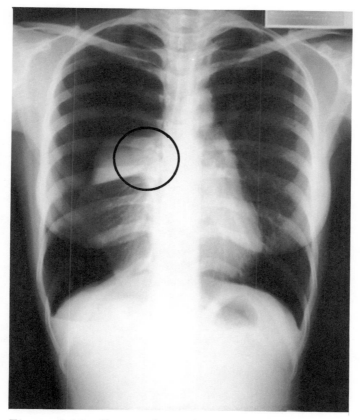

Figure 2-19. Chest radiograph of a 100% right-sided pneumothorax before insertion of chest tube. Note air bonchograms in the seventh intercostal space (circle).

The same pneumothorax is now shown with arrows demarcating the upper, lateral and lower boundaries of the collapsed right lung (Fig. 2-20).

Following the insertion of a chest tube, an AP portable radiograph was taken with the patient slightly tilted, although sitting up (note the horizontal air-fluid line in the stomach), as evidenced by the failure of the clavicles to line up perfectly (Fig. 2-21). This figure shows dramatic reexpansion of the right lung, as compared to the preceding two figures (Figs. 2-19 and 2-20). The top of the chest tube, delineated by its radiopaque line, lies at the level of the aortic arch and close to the mediastinum. Inspect the radiograph carefully and determine if reexpansion is complete, or if some of the pneumothorax persists. Once you have reached a decision, compare your results with the next figure (Fig. 2-22).

Figure 2-22 shows that a small pneumothorax persists in the superior region of the right lung, with approximately a 1.5 cm separation of the visceral and parietal pleurae, indicated by arrows in a close-up view. As previously noted, no subcutaneous emphysema can be seen, but there does appear to be fluid in the right costophrenic space. The trachea and heart are not shifted. The right border of the heart is visible again. Note the silhouette sign that occurred when the lung was collapsed and in contact with the right heart border, previously obliterating that border. The shadow of the scapulae can be seen now and could be mistaken for the edge of the pneumothorax, unless one notices the presence of tissue markings superimposed on the scapula.

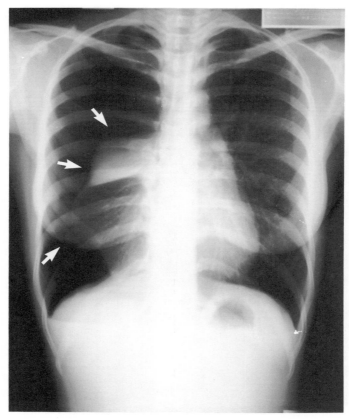

Figure 2-20. Pneumothorax. Arrows point to the boundary of the collapsed right lung.

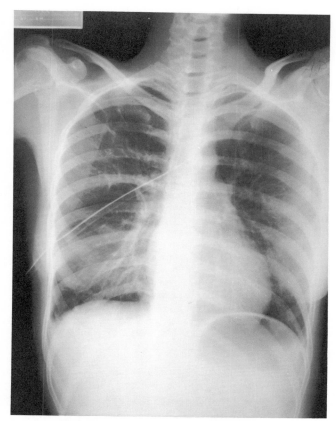

Figure 2-21. Chest radiograph taken after insertion of a chest tube, with reexpansion of the right lung.

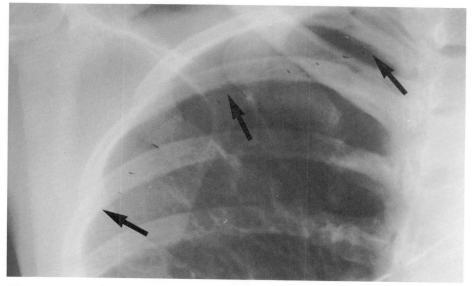

Figure 2-22. Close-up showing an unresolved pneumothorax in the right apex (arrows).

Multiple Rib Fractures with Pneumothorax

Figure 2-23 is a PA radiograph of a trauma victim admitted to the emergency room. It shows that the right lung is clear and the left lung contains several abnormalities. The most obvious of these is the fracture of the fifth, sixth, seventh and eighth ribs, where displacement has occurred. The left base displays a small degree of patchy density that is consistent with the probable diagnosis of pulmonary contusion occurring in trauma. Close inspection of the left apex reveals the presence of a pneumothorax, a common abnormality with rib fractures. The trachea is probably not shifted, but it appears to be shifted because of the patient's position. This observation is based on the asymmetrical alignment of the clavicles. Also, the left costophrenic angle appears free of pleural effusion.

Arrows in *Figure 2-24* indicate the border of the pneumothorax shown in the left apex and the series of rib fractures that were previously mentioned.

A closer view of the left lung without arrows is shown in *Figure 2-25*, giving a good view of both pneumothorax and rib fractures.

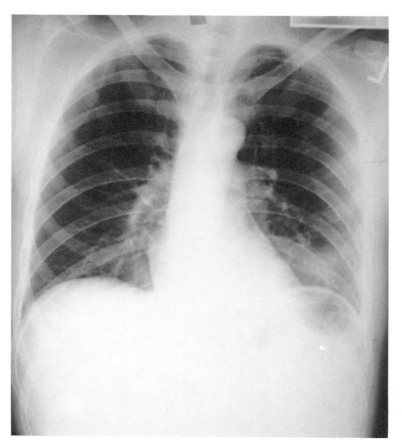

Figure 2-23. PA chest radiograph of a trauma victim, showing rib fractures and a pneumothorax.

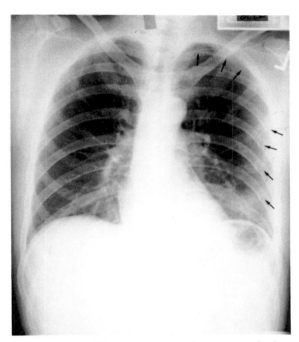

Figure 2-24. Trauma victim. Arrows mark the pneumothorax and rib fractures.

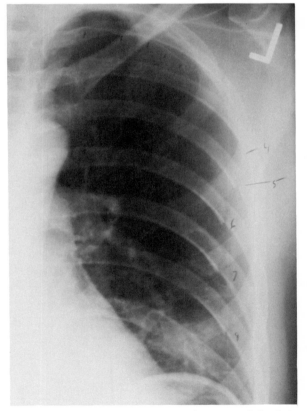

Figure 2-25. Trauma victim. Close-up of the left lung, without arrows.

Platelike Atelectasis

A classic example of platelike atelectasis is shown in the PA radiograph in *Figure 2-26*. In this radiograph, which is somewhat underexposed, long, thin densities, both horizontal and diagonal, are scattered over the lower portions of both lungs. The costophrenic angles are obscured by breast shadows. The degree of inspiration is not particularly good; the diaphragm can be seen at about the ninth rib level posteriorly. You may recall that the normal adult respiratory level is between the ninth and eleventh ribs posteriorly. The linear densities represent airless, collapsed lung tissue. An arrow marks an especially noticeable band of atelectasis in the right lower lung field.

A close-up view of the atelectasis in the base of the right lung clearly shows the linear appearance of the densities (*Fig. 2-27*). The similarity of the densities to dinner plates stood on edge is the source of the descriptive term "platelike."

The same patient shown in *Figures 2-26 and 2-27* appears in a lateral radiograph, *Figure 2-28*. Again, streaks of linear density are noted, especially toward the bases of the lungs, from anterior to posterior. The broad band of atelectasis shown in *Figure 2-26*, is again marked by an arrow. It extends from near the anterior surface of the lung toward the posterior for 2 to 3 cm before being lost to view. If one combined the PA and lateral radiographs to locate this band within the chest, the band could be placed in the right middle lobe, medial segment.

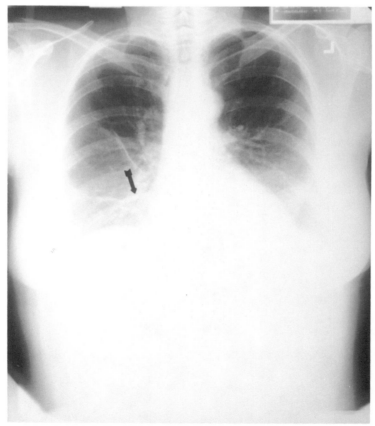

Figure 2-26. PA chest radiograph showing atelectasis in the base of the right lung (arrow).

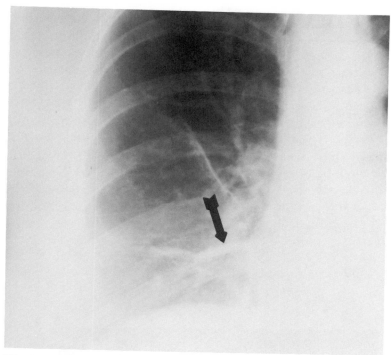

Figure 2-27. Close-up of atelectatic area.

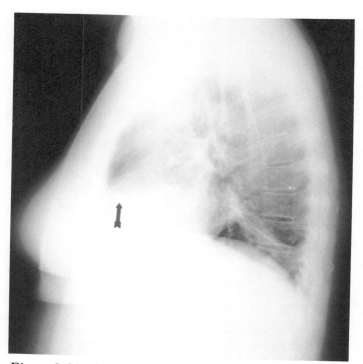

Figure 2-28. Appearance of the band of atelectasis (arrow) in a lateral radiograph.

Right Middle Lobe Pneumonia

The PA radiograph in *Figure 2-29* reveals a dense, consolidated infiltrate in the right lung. This is a classic image of a right middle lobe pneumonia. Even in the PA radiograph, the middle lobe involvement can be differentiated from the superior segment of the lower lobe by the silhouette sign (obliteration of the right heart border, indicating that the lobe is contiguous to the heart border). Normally, only the right middle lobe is next to the heart at this point in the chest.

Figure 2-30 is a lateral radiograph showing the same infiltrate as in *Figure 2-29*. It clearly demonstrates which lobe is involved, providing a classic outline of the wedge-shaped right middle lobe. Note that the infiltrate reaches to the pleural surface, although no effusion can be seen. *Figures 2-29 and 2-30* provide an excellent opportunity to practice *depth perception*, determining how deep within the lung the infiltrate is by looking at it laterally. While the obliterated right heart border is a good indicator of middle lobe involvement, it is possible for improper exposure to mask the heart border, even with right lower lobe (superior segment) infiltrates. The silhouette sign is diagnostically only as good as the overall quality of the radiograph.

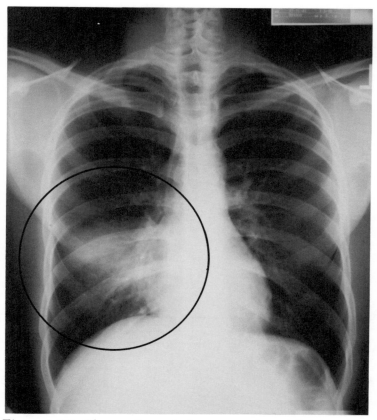

Figure 2-29. Chest radiograph showing a right middle lobe pneumonia (circle). Note silhouette sign indicating that the lobe is contiguous to the right heart border (within circle).

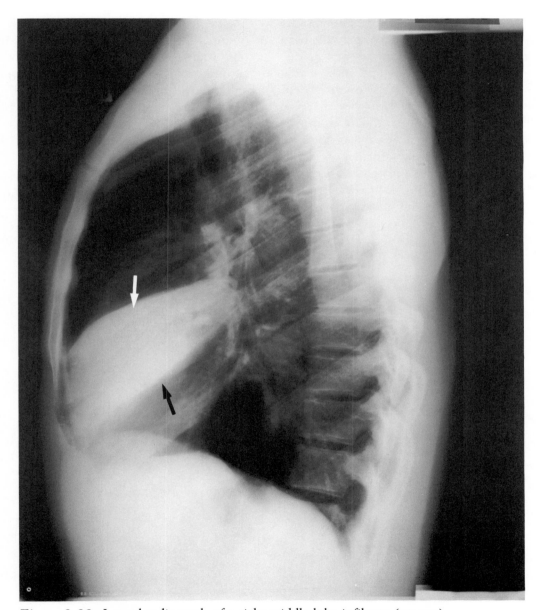

Figure 2-30. Lateral radiograph of a right middle lobe infiltrate (arrows).

Left Lung Pneumonia with Cavitation

The PA radiograph in *Figure 2-31* is of a patient diagnosed as having a left upper lobe pneumonia. Densities or infiltrates in the left upper lung field are evident, although the right lung appears clear. The density in the left lung is not immediately striking because the film is slightly overexposed, as indicated by the clear view of the vertebrae through the cardiac shadow and the much darker appearance of the right lung. The value of comparing the symmetry of right and left sides is evident here; the amount of density in the left lung can only be realized by comparing it to the even darker right lung. In addition to the infiltrate, a cavitation, or a round area of radiolucency, is seen at the level of the fourth rib posteriorly. (Find this site before proceeding.)

The cavity mentioned is outlined in *Figure 2-32* with arrows to demarcate its position. The cavity is actually air-filled, and its appearance is caused by the denser, consolidated, surrounding lung tissue. A cavity, or process of cavitation, can be thought of as a spherical structure. When this sphere is filled with air, the edge-on sides of the sphere appear whiter, because they are denser than the facing surface of the sphere, which has a hollow interior. Cavities may also be fluid-filled or display an air-fluid level. Both types of cavities can be caused by infection and a defense process that surrounds the area of infection with granulomatous tissue.

Despite the infiltrates seen on the left side, both costophrenic angles are clear. The air-fluid line in the stomach is quite noticeable (arrow), confirming the patient's upright position.

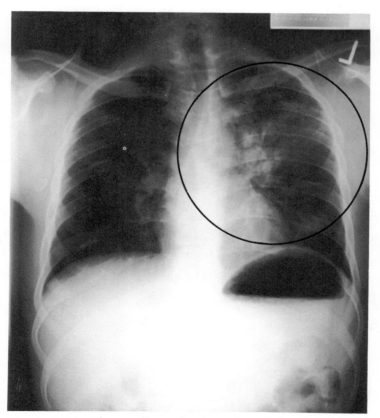

Figure 2-31. Chest radiograph of a patient with a diagnosis of left upper lobe pneumonia (circle).

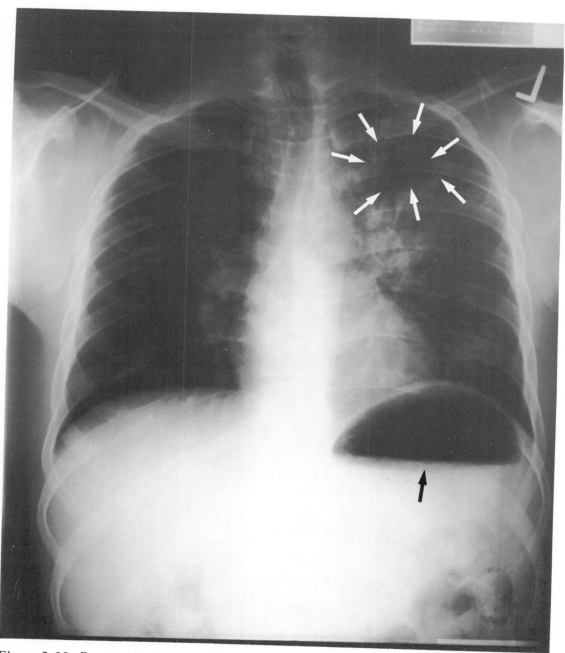

Figure 2-32. Pneumonia. Arrows indicate a cavity caused by consolidation of surrounding lung tissue in the left upper lobe.

A lateral radiograph of the same patient (*Fig. 2-33*) helps to pinpoint the position of the pneumonia in the left upper lobe. The radiograph points to the definite involvement of the apical-posterior and anterior segments of the upper division of the left upper lobe. The oblique or major fissure is well outlined by the consolidated lung tissue in the left upper lobe. Careful inspection reveals the doughnut-shaped density seen in the PA radiograph within the consolidated tissue, just anterior to the vertebrae near the top of the lung field.

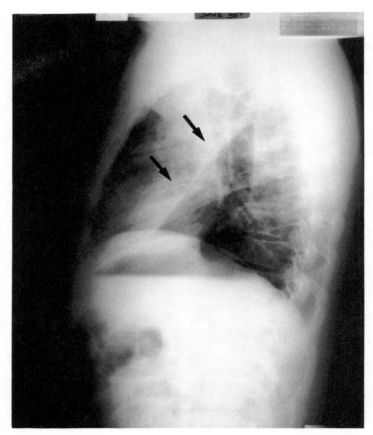

Figure 2-33. Lateral radiograph of a patient with a left upper lobe pneumonia, showing an oblique fissure (arrows).

Left Upper Lobe Pneumonia

In *Figure 2-34*, a PA radiograph was obtained of a patient with symptoms and other physical findings of a pulmonary infection. This radiograph shows a large, unmistakable, patchy density throughout a fair portion of the left lung. This, in fact, represents the appearance of a pneumonia involving the left upper lobe, primarily the anterior (upper division) segment, and the lingular division. The density has both linear and fuzzy (cloudy) appearances, indicating interstitial, as well as alveolar, involvement. Typically, interstitial fluid appears more linear, whereas alveolar filling gives a fine, fluffy and more rounded appearance. No cavitation appears within the dense area. Streaky densities are seen in the bases of both lung fields, with what may be platelike atelectasis present in the tenth intercostal space on the right side, near the right heart border. The costophrenic angles remain clear. The general appearance of the lungs shows that the diaphragm is very low, well below the eleventh rib posteriorly, and the diaphragmatic surfaces display some flattening and interdigitation. This is more pronounced in the left hemidiaphragm than in the right. Due to the low diaphragm, the heart appears elongated and narrow.

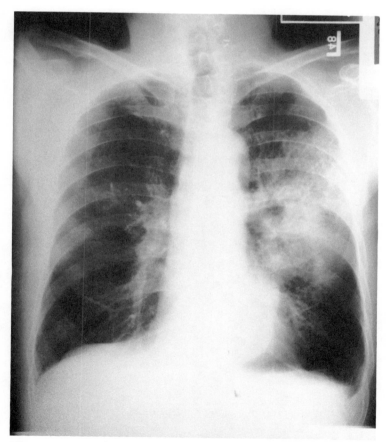

Figure 2-34. Chest radiograph of a second patient with a left upper lobe pneumonia.

83

Generalized Gram-Negative Pneumonia

It has been stressed in Part One that the chest radiograph is more descriptive than diagnostic, although additional clinical knowledge usually rules out some causes of abnormalities in favor of others. In the case presented in *Figure 2-35*, the radiograph alone could not reveal the patient's true condition without additional clinical information. The AP, semierect radiograph shows that extensive alveolar and interstitial infiltrates are present throughout both lung fields. The costo-phrenic angles cannot be seen well because of the AP position. Despite typical magnification from the AP projection, the cardiac shadow may be moderately enlarged. Without other information and from the radiograph alone, one could reasonably suspect cardiogenic or extracardiac pulmonary edema (e.g., ARDS) or overwhelming pneumonia. A differential diagnosis is not possible. The radiologist's report simply suggests all three possibilities.

The patient in this case was immunosuppressed, and was the victim of an overwhelming, opportunistic, gram-negative pneumonia that killed him. The radiograph does not show an endotracheal tube, although chest EKG leads are visible.

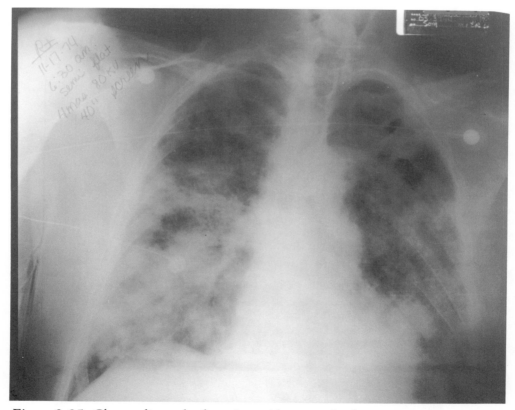

Figure 2-35. Chest radiograph of a patient with a generalized gram-negative pneumonia.

Congestive Heart Failure

The appearance of congestive heart failure, or left ventricular failure, is basically one of cardiogenic pulmonary edema. As a result, the following characteristics may be found in a chest radiograph: cardiac enlargement, with an increased C-T ratio; fluffy alveolar or linear interstitial infiltrates in the lungs; engorgement and increased prominence of the pulmonary artery in the hilar area; and increased lymphatic markings, which sometimes yield the so-called Kerley B lines. Recall that there is a similarity of appearance between the normal *expiratory* radiograph and heart failure. Knowing how the radiograph was taken and the clinical history of the patient helps in differentiating the normal expiratory appearance from heart failure. Kerley B lines (also called **linear shadows**) are an abnormality that may be seen in cardiogenic pulmonary edema. They are transverse lines up to an inch long in the lung bases that may extend to the pleura. They are actually engorged pulmonary lymphatics, not usually visible in a radiograph, that conform to the interlobular septa. When the lymphatics can no longer drain excess fluid in the interstitial space, pulmonary edema results, and the lymphatics themselves may become visibly dilated. Kerley also distinguished two other types of linear shadows, termed A and C lines, that are caused by lymphatic dilation.

The radiograph in *Figure 2-36* presents a typical picture of moderate to severe congestive heart failure. The figure is an AP portable chest radiograph of a 71-year-old male who was admitted with congestive heart failure. As is the case in many portable radiographs, the patient's position is not perfectly aligned. The patient was in a semi-upright position at the time the radiograph was made. Scapular shadows are difficult to see, but may be traced over the left lung, which is clearer than the right.

This particular radiograph shows the classic sign of heart failure in the enlarged cardiac outline; however, it should be noted that some magnification is caused by the AP position, as discussed in Part One. The clinical findings in this patient confirmed congestive heart failure. Engorgement of hilar vasculature can also be seen in both the right and left hila. The presence of pulmonary edema, particularly alveolar patterns, is more evident in the right lung than in the left. There may be atelectasis in the area of the right middle lobe. The costophrenic angles look clear, and no air bronchogram is visible.

Despite aggressive treatment, including ventilatory support with positive end expiratory pressure (PEEP), the patient relapsed, could not be weaned from the ventilator and died. An endotracheal tube, ventilator tubing and EKG monitor leads are identifiable in *Figure 2-36*.

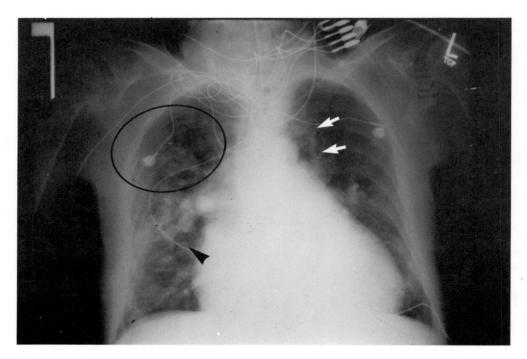

Figure 2-36. Appearance of congestive heart failure in a chest radiograph. Also, note engorgement of hilar vasculature (arrows), alveolar patterns (circled in right lung), and possible atelectasis in the area of the right middle lobe (arrowhead).

Adult Respiratory Distress Syndrome (ARDS)

A chest radiograph of a patient with adult respiratory distress syndrome (ARDS) is presented in *Figure 2-37*. Prior to inspecting the chest radiograph, a brief review of the radiologic appearance of ARDS may be useful. ARDS is produced by a number of causes, including chest trauma, high alveolar oxygen tensions and shock. The pathology ultimately involves pulmonary edema caused by increased alveolocapillary permeability and filling of the alveoli with fluid. This is, however, noncardiogenic pulmonary edema, an important fact to remember in understanding the appearance of ARDS in a chest radiograph.

If a patient has normal lungs prior to pulmonary insult, a chest radiograph will appear clear during the initial injury. Between 12 and 24 hours following the insult, fine infiltrates appear, caused by perivascular fluid accumulation and interstitial edema. This is the early appearance of ARDS in the chest radiograph. As the pulmonary edema that is characteristic of ARDS progresses over the next 12 to 24 hours, the chest radiograph shows diffuse alveolar and interstitial infiltrates, and a normal cardiac silhouette and cardiothoracic (C-T) ratio.

Figure 2-37 is an AP radiograph, which should not be unexpected considering the diagnosis and the degree of invasive maintenance that is evident. The overall appearance throughout the lung fields shows diffuse congestion, more alveolar than interstitial (note the cloudier, less linear nature of the infiltrates). The generalized whiting-out is combined with a normal C-T ratio, taking AP magnification into account. This aids in confirming noncardiogenic pulmonary edema. Left heart failure resulting in pulmonary congestion would usually yield an enlarged heart shadow, radiographically, because of inadequate emptying of the ventricles. The costophrenic angles are not clear as a result of congestion or pleural fluid. The appearance of the lungs confirms the later phase of pulmonary edema that occurs with ARDS.

In addition to being familiar with the appearance of the lungs in ARDS, the practitioner should be able to readily distinguish all other shadows from invasive lines. These lines include the following: the central venous pressure (CVP) line, marked with arrows in *Figure 2-37*, which originates on the right side and descends to near the eighth rib posteriorly (arrow); the endotracheal tube, with a clearly visible radiopaque line and a tip that is resting at the fifth intercostal space; and the monitoring electrocardiogram (EKG) leads, two of which are visible. The carina is evident and is marked by an arrow, allowing the viewer to evaluate the distance from the tip of the E-T tube to the carina.

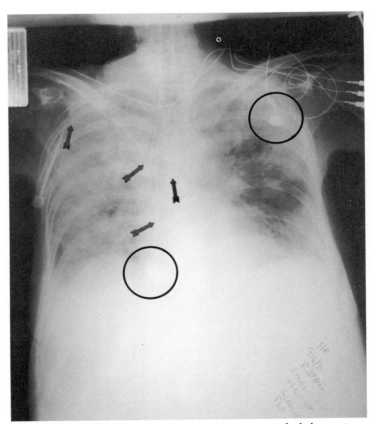

Figure 2-37. Chest radiograph showing a case of adult respiratory distress syndrome (ARDS). The three arrows on the viewer's left trace the CVP line. A fourth arrow indicates the carina. Two EKG electrodes are evident (circles).

ARDS: Ventilator Patient with Shock Lung

Figure 2-38 is an AP portable radiograph of a patient being supported on a ventilator. The patient was supine when the radiograph was made. Accordingly, the technical quality of this radiograph is not as good as an AP upright radiograph; however, the degree of inspiration is good (level of the eleventh rib posteriorly) and could have been affected by the ventilator (the presence of which is evident from the corrugated tubing visible over the left lung field). Beginning with the mediastinal area, the cardiac contours are not well defined or sharply delineated. The lung fields display a diffuse infiltrate that is more alveolar (puffy, cloudy) than interstitial (linear) in appearance. Such an image may indicate congestive heart failure; however, despite the AP magnification, the heart does not appear enlarged. In fact, the patient in this case was suffering from shock lung,

or ARDS. *Figure 2-38* is a good example of a chest radiograph characteristic of the later phase of ARDS.

In this figure, the costophrenic angle is clear on the right, but fluid shows on the left. Other shadows, not anatomical in nature, indicate the type of monitoring and critical care maintenance the patient was receiving. The use of continuous ventilation has already been noted, and the endotracheal tube is visible. The tip of the E-T tube and the level of the carina are both marked with arrows, showing good tube placement. Another radiopaque line running vertically marks a nasogastric tube (NG). A Swan-Ganz catheter is coiled over the right hilar area (SG). The tip is at the level of the sixth rib posteriorly, and the catheter advances into the pulmonary artery. A central venous line appears in the left apical region, crossing the posterior shadows of the second, third and fourth ribs before being lost in mediastinal shadows (CVP). The vertical line over the left lung field is from an EKG monitor lead (E), although the electrode cannot be seen. A similar lead extends horizontally above the right apex (E).

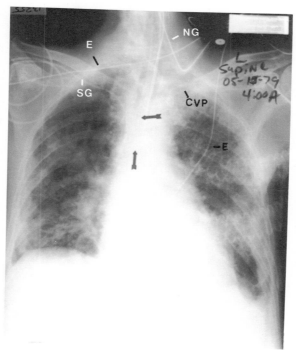

Figure 2-38. Radiograph showing shock lung, which is a form of ARDS.

89

Classic Chronic Obstructive Pulmonary Disease (COPD)

The patient with chronic obstructive lung disease has one of the most common types of adult pulmonary disease. Technically, chronic obstructive pulmonary disease is a syndrome consisting of emphysema, bronchitis, asthma and bronchiectasis in adults, with additional complications of cystic fibrosis in the pediatric and young adult group. Typically, the older patient with COPD has emphysema or bronchitis, or a mixture of these two diseases. Both are diseases of the airways. Bronchitis involves obstruction caused by increased mucus production, with mucus gland hypertrophy (increased Reid index > .36). Emphysema is a condition of the lung in which the air spaces distal to the terminal bronchioles are abnormally enlarged with destructive loss of tissue. Both conditions cause expiratory obstruction with air trapping. Advanced pulmonary emphysema shows certain radiologic changes, which, while admittedly variable among individual patients (e.g., degree of radiolucency), can be taken together to form a typical radiographic picture of emphysema.

Such is the case with the PA chest radiograph shown in *Figure 2-39.* The clinical diagnosis is advanced COPD, primarily emphysema. In this figure, the diaphragm, seen below the level of the eleventh rib posteriorly, lacks the smooth, dome-shaped appearance that is usually seen. The cardiac shadow is elongated and the aortic arch is predominantly visible, but these observations alone do not constitute abnormality. Often the heart appears elongated on deep inspiration. Regarding the lung fields, there may be some increased radiolucency, or hyperlucency, noted bilaterally in the lower lung fields. This is accentuated by overexposure, evidenced by the visibility of the vertebral column through the entire length of the cardiac shadow. Again, as a single finding, radiolucency is variable. It depends on the patient's individual body build (amount of fat, chest muscle development); technical factors, such as film exposure and processing; as well as overinflation and tissue loss. Whether the intercostal spaces are wider with severe obstructive disease is questioned by many physicians. It is probably far better to look for asymmetry rather than to try to judge whether the spaces are absolutely wider in an individual radiograph. In a fluoroscopic examination involving obstructive disease, diaphragmatic excursion may be limited because the patient breathes closer to total lung capacity than normal; however, as a static view, the PA radiograph cannot show this and resolve the question of whether the diaphragm is normally low on inspiration or abnormally low as a result of expiratory air trapping. In very thin persons, the diaphragm is commonly lower and flatter; occasionally, muscle-rib or phrenocostal attachments give a scalloped appearance, which is known as **interdigitation.** The appearance is the same as that obtained when one pushes one's fingers into soft clay. Interdigitation of the diaphragm is a common finding in the PA chest radiograph of advanced COPD.

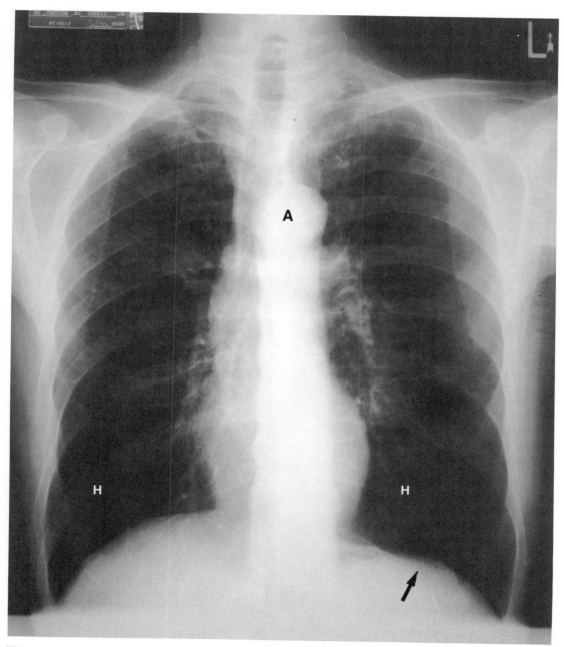

Figure 2-39. PA chest radiograph of a patient diagnosed as having advanced obstructive lung disease. The cardiac silhouette is elongated, and the diaphragms are flattened, especially in the patient's left chest (arrow). Note hyperlucent lung fields (H) and prominent aortic arch (A).

The situation is quite different in a lateral radiograph of the same patient (*Fig. 2-40*). The AP diameter is increased, and there is bowing of the sternum and an increase in the size of the retrosternal air space (the space between the sternum and the anterior border of the heart). The diaphragmatic dome appears very flat with visible attachments. There may be a greater than normal amount of kyphosis in the vertebrae. The junction of the manubrium and sternum is easily seen.

Felson (1973) summarizes the radiologic findings associated with emphysema as follows: pulmonary hyperlucency, the presence of bullae, increased AP diameter of the chest, kyphosis, anterior bowing of the sternum, increased retrosternal air space, small vertical heart, cor pulmonale, visible phrenocostal attachments, diminished diaphragmatic excursion and a low, flat diaphragm. With severe loss of the pulmonary capillary bed, causing increased pulmonary artery pressure, prominent pulmonary arteries may be seen at the hila. However, Felson cautions that many of these signs are variable and can lack reliability. He considers decreased diaphragmatic excursion, diminished vascularity of the central and peripheral portions of the lung fields (especially if coupled with enlarged hilar vessels), and retrosternal air space increase as the most reliable radiologic findings to indicate emphysema. Without fluoroscopy, diaphragmatic excursion could be seen with comparative inspiratory and expiratory PA radiographs (adding, however, to patient cost and radiation exposure). Diaphragmatic excursion is better ascertained by a chest physical examination.

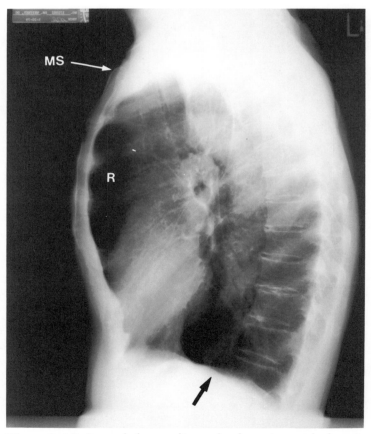

Figure 2-40. Lateral chest radiograph of a patient with chronic obstructive pulmonary disease (COPD). Note the increased retrosternal air space (R) and flat diaphragms (arrow). The junction of the manubrium and the sternum is marked (MS). Note that the AP diameter of the thorax is abnormally large.

Right Upper Lobe Bulla

Many radiographs taken of critically ill patients or those who have a history of lung disease indicate more than one abnormality. This is certainly the case in *Figure 2-41*, in which arrows indicate the approximate borders of a large right upper lobe bleb or bulla. The bulla is actually a large saclike structure with no lung tissue—a sort of giant air bubble in the lung. This lack of tissue is the identifying mark on the radiograph. The practitioner should immediately note the absence of lung tissue markings that are evident elsewhere. The portion of the bulla over the fourth intercostal space displays this tissue absence well, being perfectly clear and free of markings.

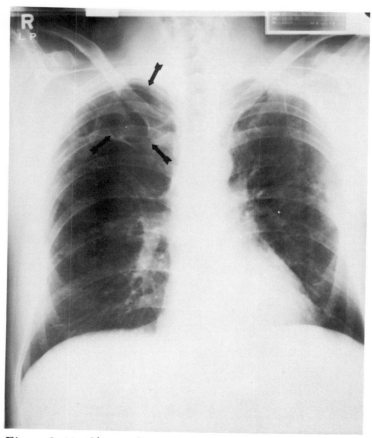

Figure 2-41. Chest radiograph showing a large right upper lobe bulla.

A close-up of the emphysematous bulla shown in *Figure 2-41* is presented in *Figure 2-42*. Bullae such as this, and smaller, superficial sacs termed blebs, are frequently noted in emphysema patients. They result from the progressive loss of lung tissue and air trapping that occurs in the disease process. Radiographically, a bulla may differ from a cavity (previously discussed in conjunction with pneumonia) by having a less well-defined and more irregular border. This appearance is caused by the pathology of the process: a bulla, as described above, is not an infectious process with granulomatous formation and, consequently, lacks the dense border that often occurs with a cavity. Compare the radiographic appearance of the bulla in *Figure 2-42* to the cavitation shown in *Figure 2-32* to distinguish the two.

A lung ventilation scan, shown in *Figure 2-43*, is compatible with the finding of a large upper lobe bulla. This case was used in Part One to exemplify the principle of ventilation scanning with radionuclides (see section entitled "Radionuclide Perfusion and Ventilation Scans"). Those basic principles should be reviewed at this point if the lung scan in *Figure 2-43* is not well understood.

Note the asymmetry between the right and left lungs on the ventilation scan. The right lung is on the viewer's left. To obtain a ventilation scan, the patient inhales a radioactive gas, xenon-133, which acts as a tracer during its movement into the lung. There is an obvious lack of ventilation in the right apical area, corresponding to the area of the bulla. Bullae often connect to patent bronchioles, but the gas exchange is usually poor and, at times, a check-valve mechanism may lead to hyperinflation and an eventual pneumothorax. The poor ventilatory exchange is well confirmed in this scan.

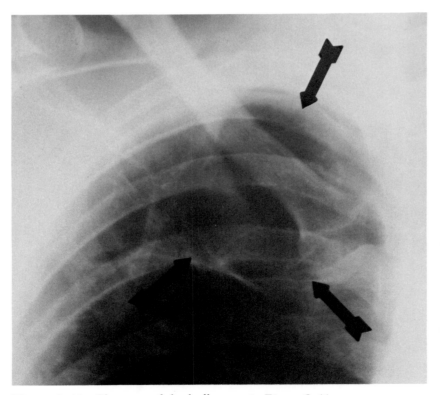

Figure 2-42. Close-up of the bulla seen in Figure 2-41.

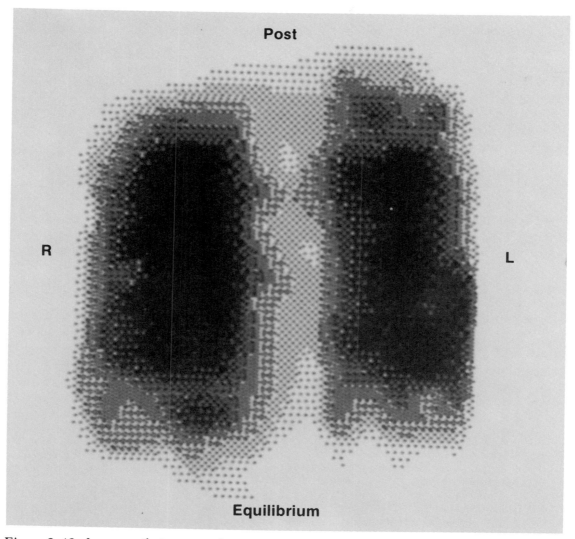

Figure 2-43. Lung ventilation scan of a patient with a right upper lobe bulla. The right lung is on the viewer's left.

Miliary Tuberculosis

No presentation of pulmonary abnormalities seen in chest radiographs would be complete without a case of pulmonary tuberculosis. However, the type of case shown in *Figure 2-44* is more interesting than a chest radiograph showing a nodular tubercle, calcified or granulomatous densities, or even a good-sized cavity because the diffuse, reticulogranular pattern of densities spread out over both lung fields of this patient represents miliary tuberculosis.

The degree of penetration is more than adequate, with the trachea perfectly visible as a gray column. The patient is slightly tilted, the clavicles are not perfectly aligned, and the heart appears to occupy more of the right side. Two hospital gown snaps are visible, one on the right and one on the left; a third snap is lost in the density of the left hemidiaphragm. Over both lung fields there is a pattern of fine densities, which appear to increase in density toward the bases of the lungs. This pattern of densities is consistent with the vascular dissemination of the tuberculous organism and the greater perfusion of the lung bases, relative to the apices. However, the presence of chest fat or a breast mass, especially in this patient, could also cause the bases to appear lighter. A streaky line of density in the left upper lung at about the level of the aortic arch is probably the primary focus of disease after the initial infection. The right and left costophrenic angles appear to be free of fluid.

The term **miliary** is derived from the Latin *miliaris* (like a millet seed), which describes the seedlike appearance of the numerous reticular densities in miliary tuberculosis. Occasionally, a caseous tuberculosis will focus in the lung or in some other organ, such as the kidneys, bones or lymph nodes, and may rupture into a vein, allowing **tubercle bacilli** (*Mycobacterium tuberculosis*) to disseminate throughout the body, as well as throughout the lungs. Because of the systemic spread, the lungs are seeded with bacilli, causing diffuse nodules scattered over the lung fields. When this occurs, it is known as miliary tuberculosis. It is more commonly seen in infants and children after primary infection, but the disease also occurs in older groups, particularly in females. Miliary tuberculosis is usually classified as acute, subacute or chronic. Meningeal infection, or tuberculosis meningitis, often accompanies miliary tuberculosis and can readily cause death unless treated pharmacologically. Before the development of streptomycin and the tuberculostatic drugs, miliary tuberculosis was almost always fatal to the patient, usually as a result of meningeal tuberculosis. With acute miliary tuberculosis, the victim is very ill (fever, chills, sweating, weakness), and a definitive nodular appearance occurs four to six weeks after the pulmonary seeding. Symptoms of the subacute form are less obvious and include prolonged fever; however, the same radiographic findings that are seen in *Figure 2-44* may eventually develop. Multiple organ systems may also become infected, as with the acute form. Chronic miliary tuberculosis may follow a latent course and remain undiagnosed for months or years.

Radiologic examination of the chest is one of the three most valuable tools in diagnosing pulmonary tuberculosis, the other two being the tuberculin test (purified protein derivative or PPD) and bacteriologic examination.

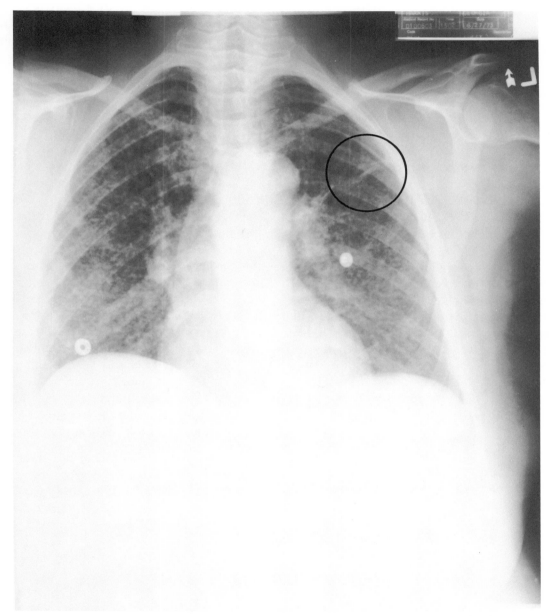

Figure 2-44. Chest radiograph of a patient with miliary tuberculosis. The streaky density in the upper left lung near the level of the aortic arch (circle) is probably the primary focus of the disease after the initial infection.

Cylindrical Bronchiectasis

The chronic disease state of bronchiectasis often produces changes in the plain chest radiograph; but, unfortunately, these changes are nonspecific. The definitive diagnosis of bronchiectasis is usually made with the use of a bronchogram, as discussed in Part One, when the clinical history is suggestive of bronchiectasis.

The term **bronchiectasis** is derived from words meaning widening of the bronchi, which is descriptive of the pathologic appearance on the bronchogram. Variations in bronchial dilation are seen with bronchiectasis, and the disease has been classified into three forms: cylindrical, saccular and cystic. When a bronchogram is performed to outline the bronchi and bronchioles, these three shapes are often distinguished. Cylindrical bronchiectasis describes a uniform expansion of the normally narrowing bronchi into a cylindrical shape. Saccular bronchiectasis refers to irregular, saclike pockets of dilation in the bronchioles, and cystic bronchiectasis is used to describe spherical dilations of the airways. The term **fusiform** refers to terminal, bulbous, spindle-shaped enlargements of bronchioles.

Bronchiectasis is usually considered to be an acquired or secondary disease state that results from chronic pulmonary infections, such as histoplasmosis, tuberculosis and others. The clinical symptoms include a productive cough with large amounts of purulent sputum. Hemoptysis may occur, and there is often a vicious cycle of recurrent respiratory infections as the disease progresses. The radiologic signs of bronchiectasis may be few. The viewer may see lung markings of increased density, such as streaky or vertical densities, extending toward the lung bases. In cases of very advanced bronchiectasis, there may be sufficient expiratory airway obstruction to cause flattening or interdigitation of the diaphragm.

Figures 2-45 through 2-49, all of the same patient, give a dramatic visual history of bronchiectasis, beginning with a standard AP portable radiograph taken in a recumbent position (Fig. 2-45), with followup bronchograms and a postoperative PA chest radiograph after a lobe was removed. In Figure 2-45, the right lung is clear and the costophrenic angle is sharply defined. In the left thorax, the dome of the hemidiaphragm and the costophrenic angle are obliterated by what may be either pleural fluid or pleural adhesions. Behind the cardiac shadow, to the left of the vertebral column, one can also discern a vertical streakiness, which is perhaps a peribronchial infiltrate. This area should be reviewed with the bronchogram in Figure 2-46 in mind. Because the patient's clinical history and symptoms, especially the existence of copious and foul-smelling sputum, pointed to bronchiectasis, a bronchogram was ordered. The bronchogram was used to evaluate the extent of pulmonary involvement and simultaneously map out areas for potential surgery, which was, in fact, performed after the bronchogram.

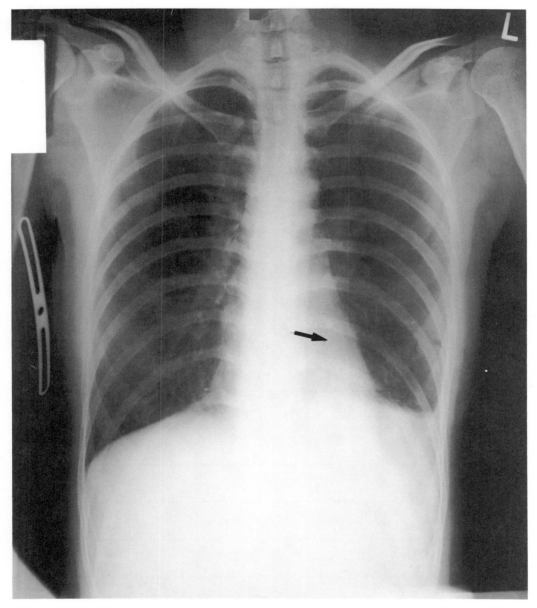

Figure 2-45. AP chest radiograph of patient with a clinical history of bronchiectasis. Note the vertical streakiness (arrow), which may be a peribronchial infiltrate.

The procedure for obtaining a bronchogram was discussed and illustrated in Part One of this text. The PA bronchogram of this patient is shown in *Figure 2-46*. Dionosil, a contrast material, was first introduced into the left side, and then into the right side to show the tracheobronchial tree, which is well outlined in *Figure 2-46*. Arrows indicate the carina and the bronchi leading to the posterior basilar segment of the left lower lobe. These bronchi are dilated and cloudy. Compare these with the clearer bronchi shown on the right side. Instead of continuing to narrow to form continually branching bronchioles, these bronchi become somewhat wider as they descend, a characteristic finding of classic cylindrical bronchiectasis. Similar changes are apparent in the anteromedial basal segment bronchi of the left lower lobe. The left hemidiaphragm is also noticeably high, with pleural fluid possibly causing obliteration of the left costophrenic angle. Compare this with the right side. Atelectasis in the left lower lobe could account for the higher hemidiaphragm. In the right lung, early changes indicative of cylindrical bronchiectasis may be present in the bronchi of the medial basal segment of the right lower lobe. The right side of the tracheobronchial tree is otherwise normal in appearance. The vertebral column is easily seen through the entire cardiac shadow.

A close-up view of several dilated bronchioles (*Fig. 2-47*) provides a good example of the appearance of bronchiectasis and its cylindrical distension.

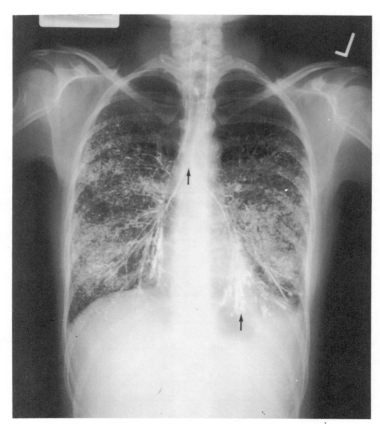

Figure 2-46. Bronchogram obtained using contrast medium in a patient with a history of bronchiectasis. Arrows indicate the carina and the bronchi leading to the posterior basilar segment of the left lower lobe.

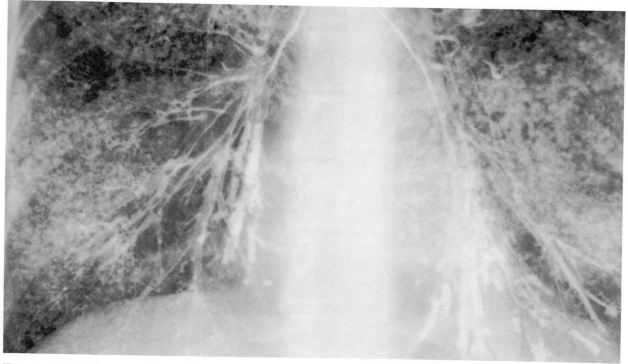

Figure 2-47. Close-up of bronchioles in the bases of lungs (seen with a bronchogram).

The PA bronchogram shown in *Figures 2-46 and 2-47* is augmented by a lateral bronchogram *(Fig. 2-48)*. The tracheobronchial tree is excellently outlined in this figure. As stressed in Part One, such outlines provided by contrast material are extremely useful learning devices for tracing the position of bronchi, which are not visible unless seen on end in standard PA and lateral chest radiographs. Compare the PA and lateral bronchograms to identify the bronchi of the posterior basal segment of the left lower lobe. An arrow marks one of the bronchi (seen previously in the PA bronchogram) that leads to the posterior basal segment of the left lower lobe. In summary, the diagnosis resulting from the bronchogram was bronchiectasis involving the posterior basal and anteromedial segments, left lower lobe and, to some extent, the medial basal segment of the right lower lobe, with the remaining lung considered normal.

Because of the atelectasis and recurrent pulmonary infection that occurred with this patient's bronchiectasis, a left lower lobectomy was performed. The bronchograms shown in this discussion were used to map out the areas of primary involvement to determine which portions of lung should be removed. The pathology report on the excised lung section showed mucus plugging and atelectasis at the base of the lobe, with a small focus of yellow, creamy, purulent material. No tumors or other abnormalities were noted. The pathologist's conclusion was that this patient had bronchiectasis with focal atelectatic areas. The radiograph in *Figure 2-49* was taken about a week after chest tubes were removed.

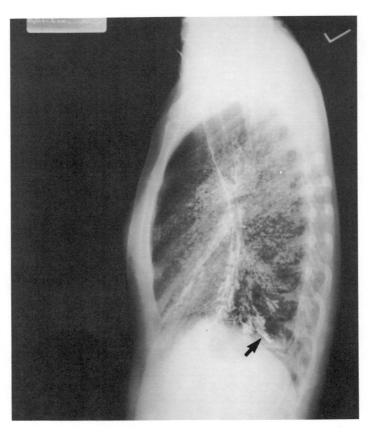

Figure 2-48. Lateral bronchogram. Note the bronchi leading to the posterior basal segment of the left lower lobe (arrow).

Figure 2-49 is a PA radiograph, although the left scapula has not been completely rotated out of view, probably because of pain and stiffness around the incision site. The sutures are clearly visible, with arrows pointing to the endpoints of the suture line. Compared to the preoperative radiograph, the left hemidiaphragm is now even higher, at the level of the tenth rib posteriorly, as a consequence of the removal of the lower lobe. There is also a small amount of fluid in the left lung base. Although the left lung is well expanded, the potential exists for residual pneumothorax, especially following the removal of chest tubes. There is, in fact, a small pneumothorax remaining in the left apex. Close inspection reveals the line of the lung border just above the third rib (posteriorly), giving approximately a 1 cm separation between the lung and the apex of the pleural cavity.

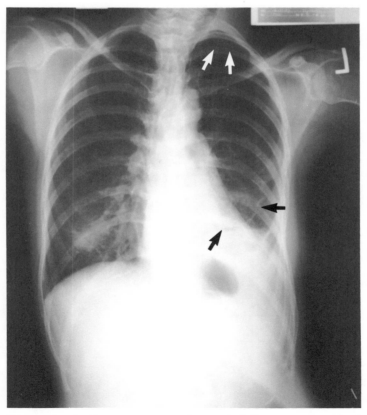

Figure 2-49. Postoperative radiograph following removal of the left lower lobe. Note the endpoints of the suture line (arrows) and the small pneumothorax in the left apex (upper arrows).

Large Right Upper Lobe Mass

The radiograph in *Figure 2-50* is both good and bad for the novice viewer. It presents an abnormality so striking that it is impossible to overlook, in contrast to those subtle abnormalities that are often a challenge to even more experienced radiologists. The radiograph is bad because it tempts the viewer to ignore a thorough and systematic review of the entire chest. The radiograph is a technically adequate PA upright. The heart and mediastinal contours are clearly visible. A large, right upper lobe mass, measuring 7 cm x 10 cm (arrows), is present, which, with the help of a lateral radiograph (not provided), is localized to the posterior segment. The margins of the mass are irregular and spiculated. Continuing with the examination, the trachea does not appear shifted, but there is a suggestion of pleural fluid in the right costophrenic angle. The patient may have had previous granulomatous inflammatory disease, as evidenced by several nodular densities in the lung fields, especially the left, at the level of the fifth rib posteriorly. The immediate suspicion is carcinoma.

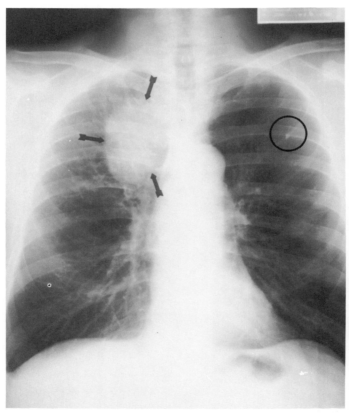

Figure 2-50. PA chest radiograph showing a large mass in the right upper lobe. Note the nodular density in the left lung field (circle).

To follow up on the mass identified on the PA radiograph, a series of tomograms was performed, four of which are reproduced in *Figure 2-51.* The location of the mass, namely the upper right chest, is shown in a sequence that begins in the upper left corner and proceeds clockwise, taking successively deeper slices through the chest. Compare the different appearances of the mass on the four tomograms.

This case is a good example of the usefulness of tomograms. Here, the tomogram allows the radi-ologist to evaluate the mass at different levels, or depths, within the chest. By doing so, a solid mass can be differentiated from one with a solid appearance that is hollow or fluid-filled. In these tomograms, no calcification or bronchi were noted. The absence of bronchial branchings (air bronchograms) indicates that the abnormal density is not restricted to parenchymal tissue alone.

The mass seen in the chest radiograph was a primary bronchogenic carcinoma, although the diagnosis was not made on the radiograph alone.

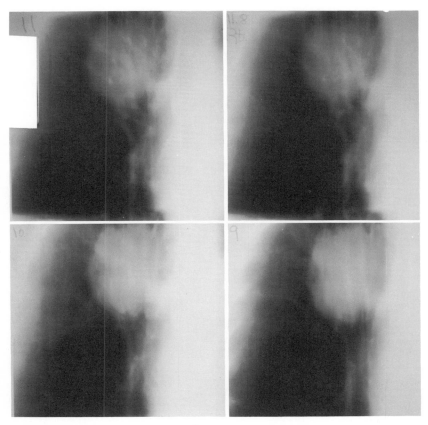

Figure 2-51. Four tomograms of a mass in the right upper lobe, arranged in clockwise order starting at the upper left.

Right Apical Nodule with Pneumonectomy

The next four figures are radiographs of the same patient. The series includes the finding of a nodule in PA and lateral radiographs, follow-up tomography, and a postoperative chest radiograph after pneumonectomy.

Figure 2-52 is a PA upright radiograph. The technical quality is quite adequate, although the patient is not perfectly positioned, as noted by the misalignment of the sternoclavicular junctions. The mediastinum, lung fields and costophrenic angles are all clear, with one exception, which will be discussed. The right hilum seems slightly elevated. Recall that, normally, the left hilum is one interspace higher than the right. Shifts in this relative positioning could be caused by atelectasis or a lesion in the left lower lobe, drawing the left hilum downward, or a similar abnormality in the right upper lobe, leading to an upward shift of the right hilum. No unusual density is apparent in the lower portion of the left lung field. Careful comparison of the right apex with the corresponding left apex shows an asymmetrical degree of density. In particular, a poorly defined area of density, 1.7 cm in size, is present, but is partly obscured by the third rib near its posterior attachment to the vertebra (arrow). This is seen only if the right and left third ribs are viewed simultaneously. The density extends slightly below the rib shadow, confirming that the density shadow is not caused by the rib. It is important to emphasize the need for bilateral comparison of the right and left sides of the chest, keeping normal anatomical differences in mind, just as with physical examination of the chest.

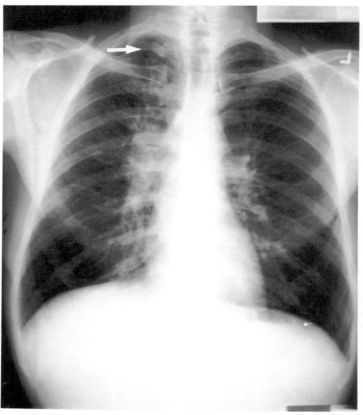

Figure 2-52. PA chest radiograph of a right apical nodule (arrow).

106

If this PA radiograph had not been so clear, a lordotic radiograph might have been obtained to further evaluate the possibility of a nodule or mass. The lordotic projection would be distinctly advantageous in this case because the suspected lesion is obscured by a rib. Recall that the tilted angle of a lordotic projection would have raised the density in relation to the third rib, which obscures it, and would have superimposed the anterior and posterior ribs and lifted the clavicles out of view. The overall effect would have been to clear out the apices for better inspection. In this case, however, tomography was chosen because there was little question that an abnormality was present.

AP tomograms obtained through the upper two-thirds of the thorax, one of which is shown in Figure 2-53, demonstrated a nodule measuring 2 cm x 1.5 cm high in the apical segment of the right upper lobe (see arrow). The mass is very irregular, with spiky margins extending outward.

The hila are well defined in this PA tomogram. The right hilum is enlarged and higher than the left, with an irregularly ovoid, 2.5 cm density on the upper margin, which is consistent with lymphadenopathy. No calcification is visible, as would be the case with histoplasmosis, which can involve calcified granulomatous infection of hilar lymph nodes. The general impression of the radiologist who reviewed this tomogram was the presence of a 2 cm nodular shadow in the right apex and associated lymphadenopathy. In such a case, bronchogenic carcinoma may be suspected.

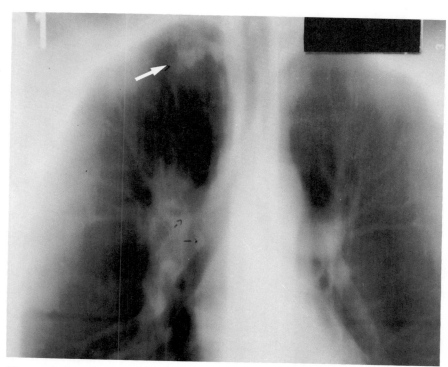

Figure 2-53. Tomogram of a right apical nodule.

Figure 2-54 is a PA upright radiograph. (How do you confirm that the patient is upright?) It was taken for follow-up after a right pneumonectomy was performed because of carcinoma in the right lung. The right hemithorax is partially filled with fluid (arrow), a normal reaction following removal of a lung. The resulting line is termed an air-fluid line. The fluid level is flat because of the presence of air; the absence of air would produce a concave meniscus. The horizontal position of the fluid line, which extends to the level of the second rib anteriorly, confirms the standing position of the patient. Sutures are visible just above the fluid, near the vertebrae (arrow). In compensation, the trachea is shifted to the right.

A lateral radiograph corresponding to the preceding PA projection is presented in *Figure 2-55*. Again, an arrow denotes the position of the air-fluid line; the sutures are visible just anterior to the arrow.

Often, information about a patient is gathered on the basis of what is not seen in a chest radiograph. In this case, without any clinical knowledge of the time these postoperative radiographs were taken, it is safe to assume that the patient was ambulatory and no longer critically maintained. This assumption is based on the absence of an endotracheal tube, chest tubes (which would be present following pneumonectomy), and chest EKG leads. The radiograph was definitely not taken in the immediate postoperative period.

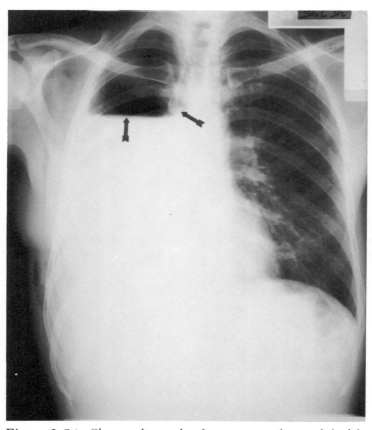

Figure 2-54. Chest radiograph of a patient with a nodule following right pneumonectomy. Note the air-fluid line (arrow on the viewer's left) and the sutures (arrow on the viewer's right), as well as the shifting of the trachea to the right.

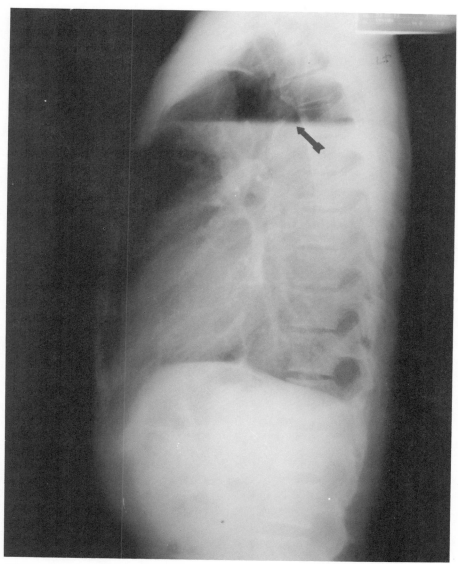

Figure 2-55. Lateral chest radiograph following right pneumonectomy.

Left Lung Peripheral Nodule

The principal comment to be made on the technical quality of the PA upright radiograph in *Figure 2-56* is that the patient is not well centered on the film plate, cutting off part of the right side and the costophrenic angle. The cardiac shadow appears to be wide, despite an adequately low diaphragm on inspiration, but the heart is within normal limits. A semicircular, upward-directed concavity of atherosclerotic plaque is visible in the aortic arch, a fairly common finding in older patients. One abnormality could be overlooked easily in the PA radiograph because of its position. Carefully follow the shadow of the third rib on the left. Before going on, determine if there is an unusual density in the shadow of this rib.

In the sixth intercostal space, indicated by arrows, a barely visible, round shadow is superimposed on the third rib's anterior shadow *(Fig. 2-57)*. This shadow could be caused by a granulomatous scar or a solitary nodule. A large blood vessel on end would not appear this far toward the periphery of the lung. Furthermore, this radiograph was taken in August 1977; the density in question was not present in radiographs taken in May 1976. Follow-up tests, such as tomography, are indicated by this finding. A biopsy of this area in the left upper lobe revealed a granular, gray-brown consolidation approximately 1.5 cm in diameter. Next to this consolidation was an area of cavitation, about 5 mm in diameter, that contained yellowish-green matter. A frozen section showed a necrotizing granulomatous site of inflammation (nonmalignant), called a caseating granuloma. The granuloma was caused by an infection from rare, acid-fast organisms. The term caseating refers to the cheeselike appearance of the necrotic tissue at the infection site.

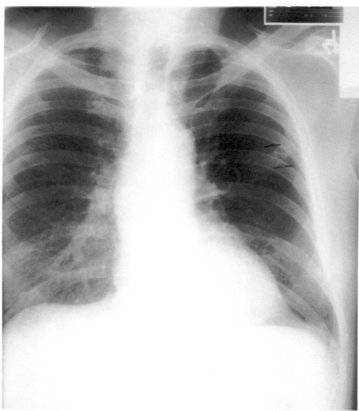

Figure 2-56. PA chest radiograph of a patient with a peripheral nodule in the left lung.

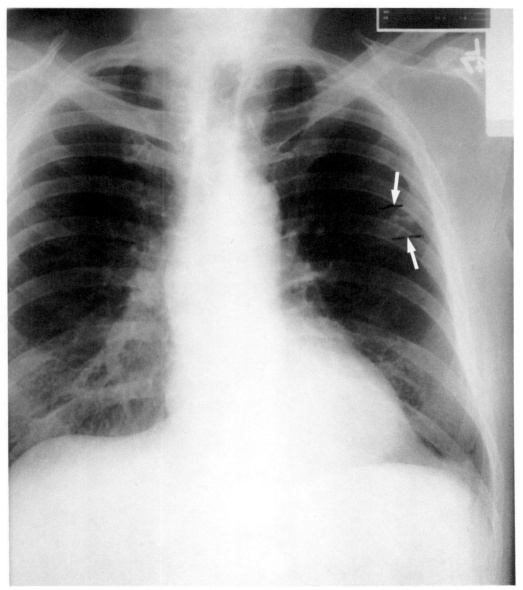

Figure 2-57. Peripheral nodules. Arrows indicate left lung peripheral nodule.

Metastasized Pulmonary Carcinoma

Figure 2-58 shows a less obvious radiographic finding of COPD deterioration in a 47-year-old male. The heart is normal in size, and the upper mediastinal contours seem normally defined. However, since a chest radiograph was taken three years earlier, a large (9 cm), irregular mass has appeared in the right upper lobe, and many smaller, ovoid nodules (5 mm to 5 cm) are scattered throughout both lungs. The pleural surfaces are currently free of fluid.

This is the appearance of widespread pulmonary metastatic disease, possibly originating from a nonthoracic source or a primary alveolar cell carcinoma in the site of the largest lesion. The diagnosis of carcinoma was confirmed by pathology following a scalene lymph node biopsy.

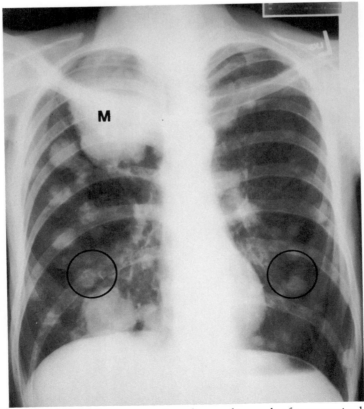

Figure 2-58. Appearance in a chest radiograph of metastasized pulmonary carcinoma. Note the large irregular mass (M) in the upper right lobe and the smaller ovoid nodules scattered through both lungs (circles).

112

Pulmonary Embolism and Perfusion Scan

The most definitive method of diagnosing a pulmonary embolism is pulmonary angiography. Although a normal lung perfusion scan can definitely rule out pulmonary emboli, an abnormal scan by itself is not diagnostic. The diagnosis of pulmonary embolism is frequently made by combining the clinical picture, history and various, less definitive laboratory data. The chest radiograph may yield variable findings with pulmonary embolism, ranging from no abnormalities to the presence of infiltrates. No infiltrates or signs of pulmonary embolism are visible in *Figure 2-59*. Under these circumstances, the perfusion scan is one of the best diagnostic procedures and may eliminate the need for angiography. This procedure, discussed in Part One, should be reviewed, if necessary.

Because decreased perfusion can be caused by a number of disease processes (asthma, COPD, pneumonia), an area of decreased perfusion is not diagnostic of pulmonary embolism. Other factors, such as history, symptoms and laboratory data, must also be considered. PA and lateral chest radiographs taken at the time of the lung scan are reviewed along with the scans. Because perfusion scans are sensitive to pulmonary emboli, a normal scan virtually rules out the possibility of pulmonary embolism. In a patient who has a normal chest radiograph and multiple perfusion defects, but who does not have lung disease, a pulmonary embolism is highly probable. If a patient without previous lung disease presents with both an infiltrate on chest radiographs and corresponding perfusion defect, the presence of *additional* perfusion defects makes pulmonary embolism *likely*. However, the diagnosis cannot be made from this test alone. In patients with existing pulmonary disease, a ventilation scan is frequently obtained and

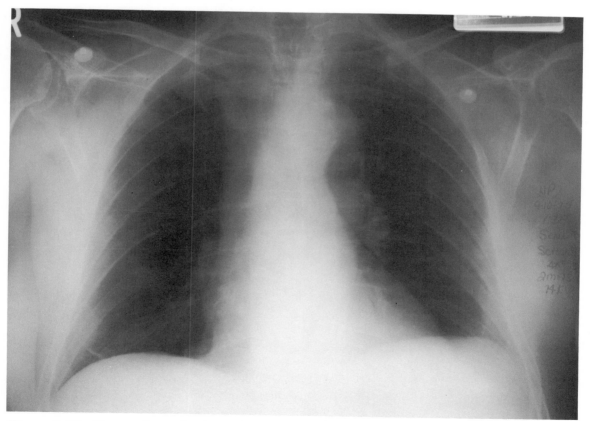

Figure 2-59. Chest radiograph, clear of infiltrates, of a case of suspected pulmonary embolism.

is compared with the perfusion scan. If the degree of perfusion defect in a given area greatly exceeds the degree of ventilation defect, a pulmonary embolism is suspected.

A negative chest radiograph does not rule out a pulmonary embolism. *Figure 2-59* is a chest radiograph of a 68-year-old male who presented at the emergency room with a sudden onset of chest pain, dyspnea and hypoxemia. Notice that the aorta is tortuous, with calcium in the distal arch. **Tortuous** is a term often used to describe a twisted, turning aortic arch. Also observe that the lung fields and pleural surfaces are clear and that no infiltrates can be seen. Except for a tortuous aorta with calcification, this radiograph is normal.

However, despite the normal chest radiograph,

a pulmonary perfusion scan showed a massive perfusion defect throughout the right lung, involving all lobes.

Figure 2-60 shows the scan from the anterior position; the right and left lungs are at the top of the figure, with the right lung appearing much lighter and, therefore, underperfused. The bottom of the left lung is also lighter in appearance than the rest of the lung field. The side view of the lung (bottom of the figure) shows the left lung, which has good perfusion, except for the lingular wedge. This observation on the lateral view corresponds well with the fainter outline of the left lung's lower portion in the anterior scanning view above it.

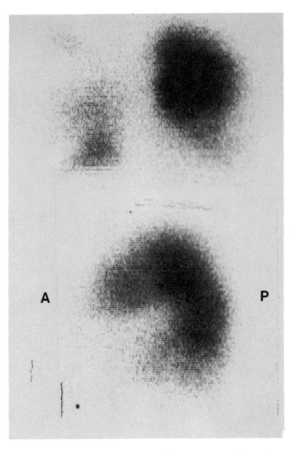

Figure 2-60. Anterior perfusion scan of a patient with a suspected pulmonary embolism. Top: right lung is on the viewer's left. Note decreased perfusion of the right lung. Bottom: lateral scan of left lung, showing good perfusion, except for lingular wedge.

Figure 2-61 again shows the results of the scan, with a posterior scan of both lungs at the top of the figure and a lateral view of the right lung at the bottom. Although scanned posteriorly, the right lung (on the viewer's left) once again appears much fainter than the left lung. Notice the difference in the lower portion of the left lung between this figure and the preceding anterior scan. Posteriorly, the bottom of the left lung is traced heavily and the lingular perfusion defect is not as evident as on the anterior scan. This is because the left lower lobe, apparently not involved, hides the lingular division, which is the lower portion of the upper lobe. (The reader may wish to review the segmental and lobar anatomy of the left lung.) Finally, the lateral view of the right lung is much lighter than the lateral view of the left lung in the preceding figure (*Fig. 2-60*), indicating decreased perfusion. The perfusion scan clearly demonstrates that a normal chest radiograph does not necessarily rule out a pulmonary embolism.

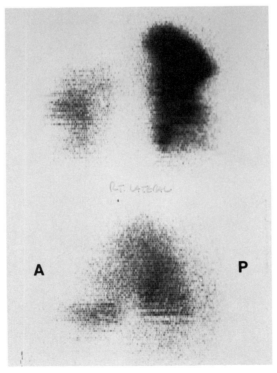

Figure 2-61. Posterior perfusion scan. The right lung is still on the viewer's left (top part of the figure). The lateral scan (bottom) is of the right lung.

Pulmonary Embolism with Pleural Effusion

Figure 2-62 is a semierect AP radiograph showing a tortuous aorta. The right lung field shows two areas of patchy consolidation. The first is in the area of the right hilum, at about the level of the seventh and eighth ribs posteriorly, while the second is in the medial right lung base (the lower portion of the lung field toward the cardiac shadow). In addition, the total obliteration of the right costophrenic angle, covering a third of the right hemidiaphragm, is a more obvious finding. The left lung is essentially clear, and what can be seen of the left costophrenic angle is also clear.

This patient did, in fact, have a pulmonary thromboembolism, and the positive findings in the chest radiograph were confirmed by lung scans. A moderate-sized pleural effusion related to the thromboembolism resulted in the right lung.

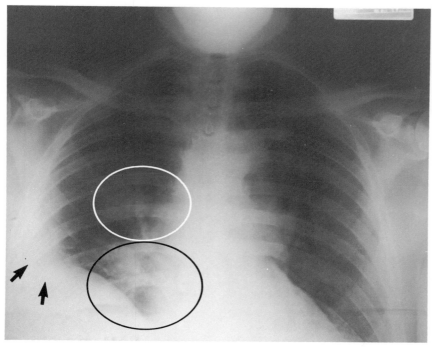

Figure 2-62. AP chest radiograph of a case subsequently confirmed as pulmonary embolism, with a large right pleural effusion (arrows). Note the areas of patchy consolidation in the right lung field (circles).

Although the lung perfusion scan is not definitive in diagnosing a suspected pulmonary embolism, such a scan can confirm the diagnosis. In the patient shown in the preceding AP radiograph (*Fig. 2-62*), anterior, posterior, right and left lateral perfusion scans were all performed following intravenous injection of a tracer material.

In both the posterior (*Fig. 2-63*) and anterior scan (*Fig. 2-64*), a large perfusion defect in the basilar segments of the right lower lobe is visible. This corresponds to the zones of patchy consolidation and pleural effusion at the right base. *Figure*

2-63 shows a posterior scan of both lungs, with the right lung on the viewer's left. There is also a segmental perfusion defect in the apical and anterior segments of the right upper lobe (see the right lateral view to localize the involved segments), which is more extensive than the patchy infiltrate in the suprahilar portion of the right lung. The right lateral scan of the right lung (bottom of the figure) clearly indicates the apical and basilar perfusion defects that were seen in the PA and AP projections.

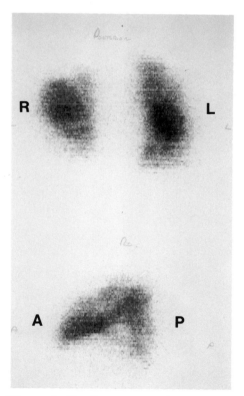

Figure 2-63. Posterior perfusion scan. The right lung is on viewer's left (top), and the lateral scan is of the right lung (bottom). Note the light areas of decreased perfusion.

The most interesting aspect of the scan in *Figure 2-64* (right lung on viewer's left) is that the lateral view of the left lung shows a large perfusion defect involving most of the posterior segment of the left upper lobe, although no infiltrate appeared in this area in the chest radiograph. This observation is further proof that a pulmonary embolism does not always result in radiographic changes. Even when there are changes, not all perfusion defects correspond one-to-one with radiographic changes. This fact is aptly demonstrated when these perfusion scans are compared with the radiograph of the same patient.

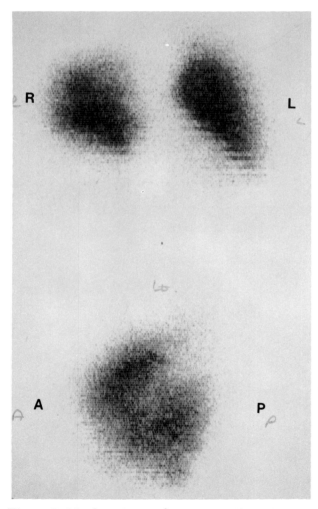

Figure 2-64. Anterior perfusion scan. The right lung is on the viewer's left (top), and the lateral scan is of the left lung (bottom).

Cystic Fibrosis

Casual inspection of *Figure 2-65* (next page) might lead the viewer to conclude that there are no abnormal findings. However, viewing the radiograph systematically, as discussed in Part One, uncovers several features. This is a radiograph of a cystic fibrosis patient admitted to the emergency room.

First, consider the technical quality of the radiograph. The patient's position is good (symmetrical clavicular position), the projection is PA (scapulae are rotated outward), and the radiograph is somewhat overexposed, allowing the vertebral column to be visible through the entire cardiac silhouette. As a result, the lung fields, in general, are relatively darker.

Systematic inspection of the entire chest reveals several features worth noting in light of the patient's history of cystic fibrosis. Increased interstitial markings of the lungs are present and are more pronounced in the mid and lower lung fields. Some streaky densities are visible in the region of the right middle lobe and left lower lobe.

These could be underestimated easily, given the degree of overexposure. No definite, discrete consolidaton is apparent, however. A slight thickening or blunting of the right costophrenic angle is also present. The anterior corner of the costophrenic angle can be differentiated from the posterior on the right side, showing the backward and downward sweep of the diaphragmatic surface. Finally, a vague, but definitely round, density is visible on the right side over the fourth rib anteriorly and the eighth rib posteriorly. This density is most probably a nipple shadow because the patient is a female. The general impression derived from this radiograph is that the patient has the chronic lung changes that occur with cystic fibrosis. There is also a possibility of bronchopneumonia in the left lower lobe and the right middle lobe. The radiograph itself is not diagnostic, but simply descriptive; that is, the streaky densities that are noted provide the appearance of bronchopneumonia. Technically, of course, only the densities and shadows on the radiograph can be described, but these are typically considered in the context of the patient's chief complaint and clinical history.

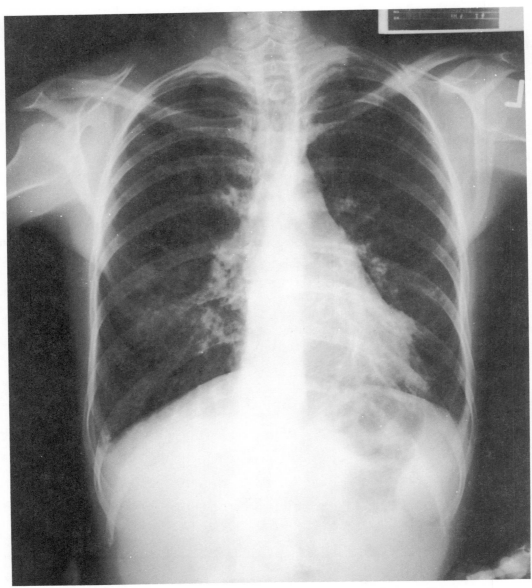

Figure 2-65. PA chest radiograph of a patient with a history of cystic fibrosis.

Pneumoconiosis

The immediate impression given by the radiograph in *Figure 2-66* is that a coarse, grainy infiltrate is diffused throughout both lungs. The left costophrenic angle is visible and appears clear. The trachea and carina are clearly visible; the carina appears at the level of the seventh rib posteriorly. The pattern of the infiltrate is considered to be both interstitial and alveolar. Recall that interstitial infiltrates are more linear in appearance, whereas alveolar filling typically gives a fine, fluffy, more rounded appearance. The right costophrenic angle is not as clear as the left; in fact, the results of a lung biopsy are visible in the right lower lobe. Even the heart borders are indistinct because of the infiltrates in the lungs. However, the heart does not appear to be enlarged; the cardiothoracic ratio is less than 50 percent. The radiologic impression is that the patient has diffuse interstitial lung disease, probably diffuse interstitial fibrosis. If the patient's history revealed a chronic condition, this radiograph could be showing pneumoconiosis, sarcoidosis, scleroderma, histiocytosis, or idiopathic interstitial fibrosis.

The pathology report on the biopsied lung material showed an almost total obliteration of normal lung tissue, with the formation of small blebs in some areas, fibrosis, and the loss of fine alveolar structure. There was extensive bronchiolar hyperplasia and marked smooth muscle hyperplasia around these bronchioles. The microscopic diagnosis was advanced diffuse interstitial fibrosis. The prognosis for this patient was very poor.

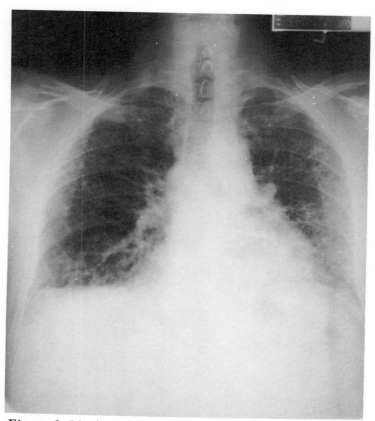

Figure 2-66. Appearance of advanced pneumoconiosis in a chest radiograph.

Histoplasmosis

Figure 2-67 is a PA radiograph of a standing patient with good position and inspiration. The radiograph has a normal degree of penetration. The obvious finding is that numerous small, round densities are scattered throughout the lungs. In addition, bilateral hilar densities are present. The scattered nodules and overall appearance of this chest are typical of histoplasmosis, although this case is more obvious than many cases because so many nodules are evident. The densities themselves are calcifications resulting from healed histoplasmosis sites. The hilar densities are enlarged and calcified lymph nodes. The organism responsible for histoplasmosis is the fungus *Histoplasma capsulatum*, which is commonly found around hay or grass clippings in rural areas in the midwestern United States and elsewhere. The radiographic findings may be confirmed by a "histo" skin test, in which a dilute solution of the organism protein is injected intradermally. If the patient has been previously infected with Histoplasma capsulatum and is immunologically competent (i.e., capable of an immune response with circulating antibodies and sensitized T lymphocytes), a reaction will occur at the skin site. This reaction is local inflammation caused by interaction between the antigenic protein and the lymphocytes (sensitized specifically to this organism during the previous infection), which seek to neutralize a new exposure to the organism. The infection is limited by the body's immune response, leaving the calcified scars seen in *Figure 2-67*, which are healed granulomas. In *Figure 2-68*, arrows point to a nodule in the right lung periphery and to a calcified, enlarged hilar lymph node in the left hilar region. This radiograph was taken in October 1975. Compared to a previous PA radiograph taken in September 1974, no changes could be observed, which is consistent with the healed and static nature of the disease. (NOTE: Although the patient's position is good in the sense that it is symmetrical, with the sternoclavicular joints aligned, the patient was not centered to the film itself).

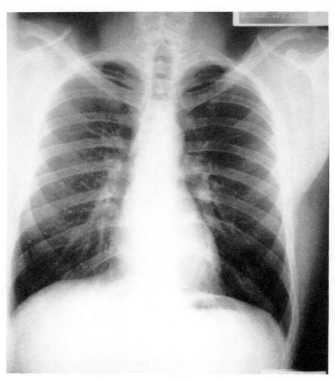

Figure 2-67. Appearance of histoplasmosis in a chest radiograph.

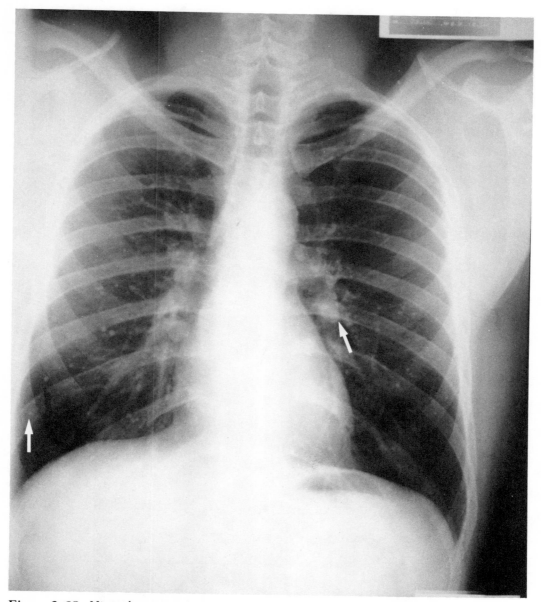

Figure 2-68. Histoplasmosis. Arrows indicate a right lung nodule and a calcified hilar lymph node in the left hilar region.

A lateral radiograph of the same patient is presented in *Figure 2-69*, showing that the calcified nodules are also present from the anterior to the posterior portions of the lung. An arrow indicates one of the many nodules that are superimposed on the cardiac shadow. The hilar lymph nodes are also very visible in this lateral radiograph.

It may be appropriate to pass along a helpful hint given by Dr. Benjamin Felson (1973) for distinguishing between a granuloma, or nodule, and a blood vessel seen end-on. This is not really a problem in the case at hand because the densities in this radiograph are numerous and are in the periphery of the lung, where sizeable blood vessels would not be found. In the case of an isolated density, however, it is often necessary to differentiate a nodule from a blood vessel.

Careful inspection of a normal blood vessel seen on end usually reveals an adjacent bronchus on end, giving two shadows side by side, which appear as so: ●○ This would not be the case with a calcified nodule or any other lesion. A good example of this normal anatomical finding is shown in *Figure 2-70*, in which the upper arrow marks a blood vessel and bronchus, side by side and seen on end. *Figure 2-71* is a close-up view that clearly shows the bronchiole and blood vessel seen on end next to each other (upper arrow). Felson refers to this as the "spectacle sign."

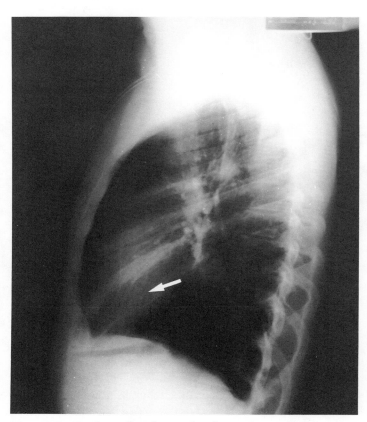

Figure 2-69. Lateral radiograph of a patient with histoplasmosis. One of the many nodules is marked (arrow).

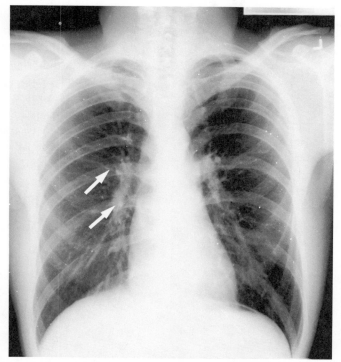

Figure 2-70. Normal chest radiograph, with a blood vessel and bronchus seen on end and side by side (top arrow).

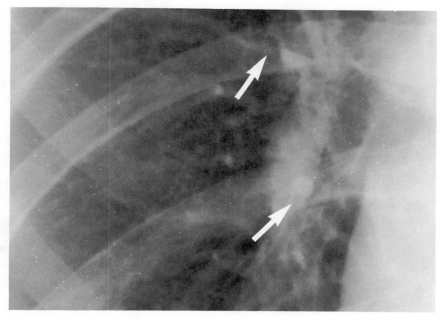

Figure 2-71. Close-up of blood vessel and bronchus seen on end. The lower arrow indicates a blood vessel with a faintly visible bronchus just above it.

Extrapleural Bleed

The patient whose radiograph is shown in *Figure 2-72* displayed symptoms of infection. A large circular density is visible in the lower right lung field. Previous decubitus projections of the patient's chest demonstrated an air-fluid level within this rounded density; the density could not be separated from the pleural surface. Tomograms were also performed and confirmed a 7 cm x 7 cm density that contained air. In light of the symptoms, a pulmonary abscess was suspected.

The right heart border has been marked by a single arrowhead in the figure. The obliterated right costophrenic angle indicates the presence of pleural effusion. In addition to the hazy density indicative of the pleural effusion in the right lower lung, a barely visible, but definite, border runs diagonally down from the right lower edge of the lung to the area of the right diaphragm (arrows), which suggests an extrapleural density. This density was caused by a large extrapleural bleed following a pleural tap to remove the effusion. This figure is an unusual example of both pleural effusion and extrapleural density.

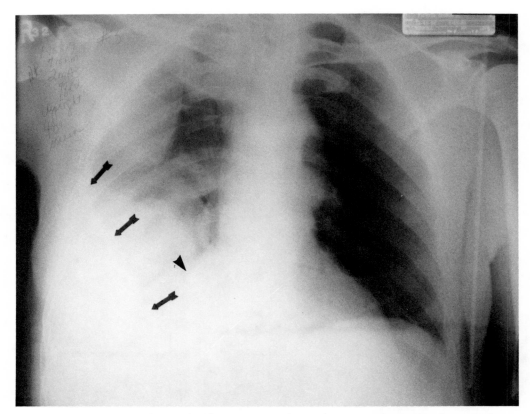

Figure 2-72. Chest radiograph of a patient with a pulmonary abscess in the right lung, extrapleural bleed (arrows), and pleural effusion.

Subdiaphragmatic Air Following Cholecystectomy

Figures 2-73 through 2-77 are of one patient who underwent a cholecystectomy a short time before the first radiograph *(Fig. 2-73)* was taken. The radiograph is slightly underexposed, although the patient's position is good, as evidenced by the alignment of the clavicles. Knowing that this patient had recently undergone abdominal surgery helped to explain the atypical findings noted on close examination of the radiograph. First, as a result of the surgery, a thin concavity of free air is visible below the right hemidiaphragm (arrows). Second, the right costophrenic angle is blunted, probably by a pleural effusion. Third, linear densities, possibly caused by atelectasis and perhaps accentuated by shallow inspiration because of pain, are evident on the original radiograph (difficult to see in the figure). These linear densities are more pronounced and noticeable in the right lung base than in the left. These three findings are all consistent with the results of abdominal surgery. Note that what might be taken for a meniscus of fluid in the left costophrenic angle is really a curved breast shadow, and the angle presents as a darker triangle below the tissue shadow. A close-up view of the subdiaphragmatic air is shown in *Figure 2-74*.

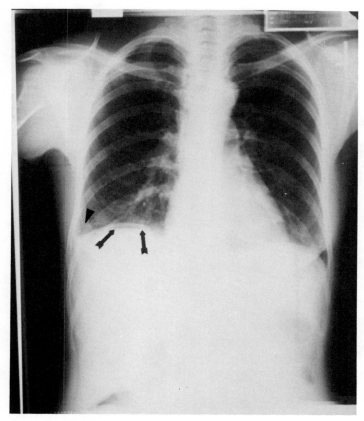

Figure 2-73. Chest radiograph showing free air under the right diaphragm (arrows) and linear densities (arrowhead).

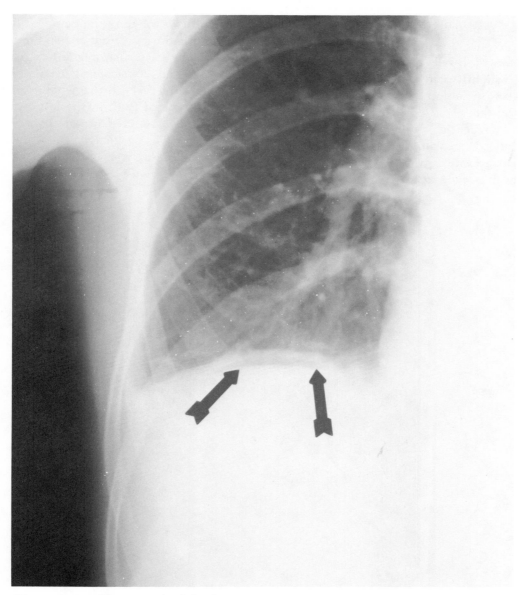

Figure 2-74. Close-up of subdiaphragmatic air.

In the lateral radiograph (*Fig. 2-75*), free sub-diaphragmatic air is again clearly visible (arrow). Even without the corresponding PA radiograph, it would be safe to conclude that the air was below the right diaphragm because the higher dome is outlined. This conclusion, of course, assumes that this patient's left diaphragm is not abnormally elevated.

The trachea is well delineated, and some branching is visible. Also, what is probably an artery on end is visible between the carinal area and the vertebrae.

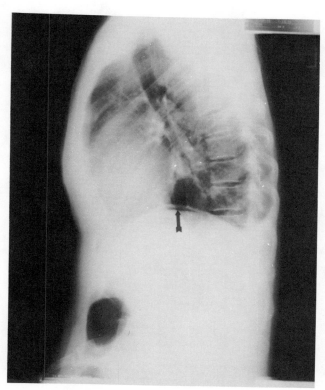

Figure 2-75. Lateral chest radiograph showing subdiaphragmatic air.

A follow-up radiograph of the patient that was taken four days later (*Fig. 2-76*) provides a good example of why viewers should always keep normal antomy in mind. After systematically inspecting the entire radiograph, two possible abnormalities can be considered. First, there is a definite nodular density over the left lower lung field (arrow), and second, the right costophrenic angle is not symmetrical with the left, suggesting partial obliteration on the right. Of course, the latter finding is the remaining, but improved, postoperative pleural effusion. Note also that the free air below the diaphragm has been absorbed. The nodular density on the left is a normal finding, representing a nipple shadow that was not seen on the previous radiograph. The level of inspiration, now at the eleventh rib posteriorly, is better than in the previous PA radiograph. The degree of penetration is also better. The close-up (*Fig. 2-77*) gives a good view of the nipple shadow and the surrounding breast shadow.

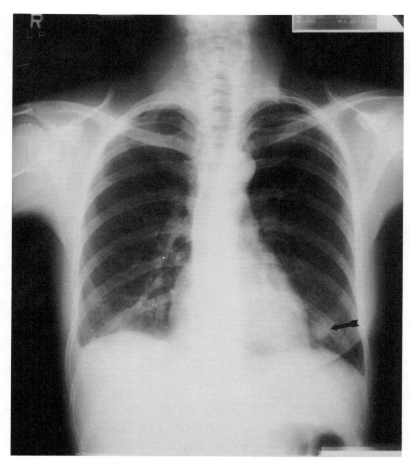

Figure 2-76. Follow-up chest radiograph showing clearance of subdiaphragmatic air, some remaining right pleural effusion, and a left nodular density (which is a nipple shadow).

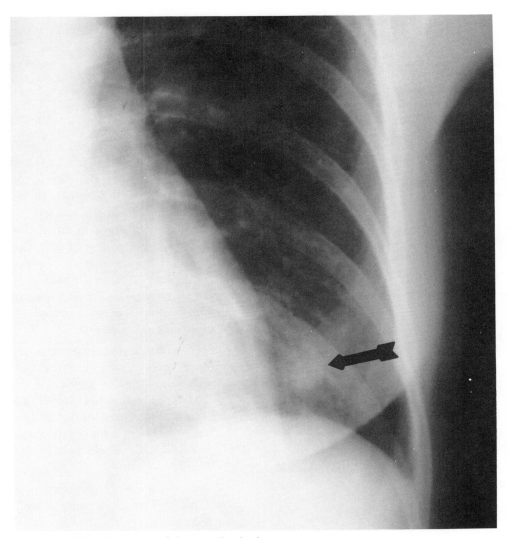

Figure 2-77. Close-up of the nipple shadow appearance.

Gunshot Victim with Extrapleural Bleed

The woman shown in the radiograph in *Figure 2-78* was the victim of a shooting that left two bullets in her chest and abdomen. Locate both metallic bullets, which are marked by an arrow. This is the same case used in Part One to exemplify an extrapleural density. Because this case has been partially presented, it is a useful tool for self-assessment. Review *Figure 2-78* carefully and try to answer the following questions:

a. Is this an AP or PA chest radiograph?

b. Is there any evidence that the patient is in an upright position?

c. What can you conclude concerning the patient's position?

d. Is the radiograph under, over or normally exposed?

e. What is the anterior rib level of the bullet on the right side?

f. What is the posterior rib level of the bullet below the diaphragm?

g. What do you think the radiopaque line is?

h. Are there any chest tubes in place?

i. To what abnormality do the other arrows point? (This is the most difficult question for the beginner.)

j. Are the right and left lungs symmetrically radiolucent?

Here are the answers:

a. AP (Note the scapular shadows, more visible on the right.)

b. No, since no air-fluid line can be seen in the stomach

c. Would you still be on your feet after being shot twice? She is almost certainly supine or semirecumbent.

d. Overexposed (Note the appearance of bones in the chest.)

e. Fifth rib anteriorly

f. Twelfth rib posteriorly

g. A nasogastric tube

h. No, this radiograph was taken to determine the degree of trauma prior to placing chest tubes.

i. This is an example of an extrapleural density, with the density in this case created by blood. Note the classic appearance of an extrapleural density that is exemplified here—namely, the sharp, well-defined border projecting in from the chest wall. This can be compared with the fuzzier, less defined appearance of a pleural effusion. The blood seen in the radiograph is outside both visceral and parietal pleurae (See the Part One section entitled "Pleural and Extrapleural Lesions.").

j. No, despite the overexposure, the right lung looks denser because of the presence of fluid in the posterior pleural space (The patient is not standing up, so fluid can accumulate around the lung.). The air-filled left lung is more radiolucent. The right costophrenic angle is obliterated by this fluid.

Figure 2-79 gives a close-up view of the extrapleural bleed in the right chest, as well as the bullet near the seventh rib.

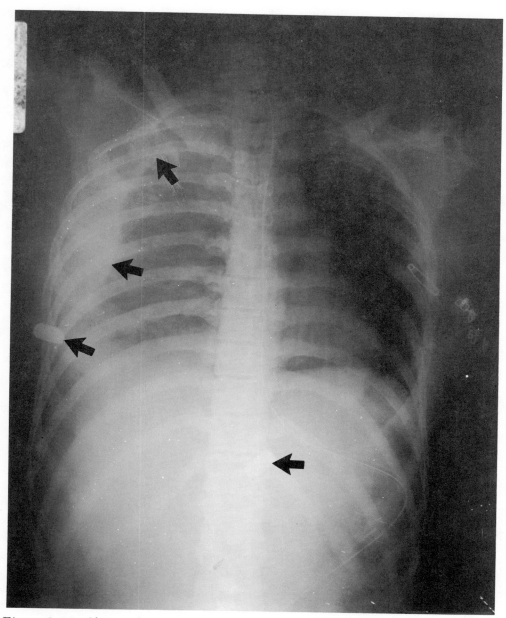

Figure 2-78. Chest radiograph of shooting victim with resulting extrapleural bleed on the right.

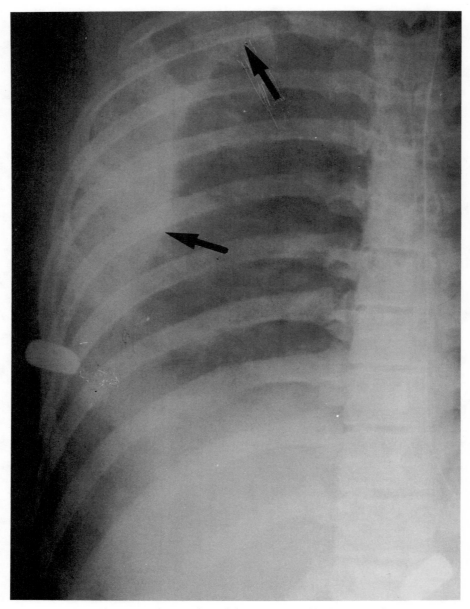

Figure 2-79. Close-up of extrapleural density caused by bleeding from the chest wall.

EPILOGUE

Parts One and Two of this text on chest radiographs have served complementary functions. Part One provided the basic skills necessary for the clinical use of chest radiographs in evaluating patients. These skills encompassed a framework of terms and principles essential to understanding radiographs and a specific system for approaching each chest radiograph. A systematic method of reviewing chest radiographs was stressed, a method that should become a habit with anyone who sees radiographs frequently. The conceptual groundwork laid in Part One was applied to actual clinical cases in Part Two. The cases in Part Two also offered radiographic examples of common chest pathologies.

This text must, of necessity, have a Part Three, which can only be written by the reader and, in fact, *must* be written by the reader if Parts One and Two are to prove useful. This last part is the continued practice in applying the principles presented here. The best way to use the concepts and examples that have been provided in this text is to look at radiographs as often as possible with information provided by the radiologist's report, and with background clinical knowledge of the patient whenever possible. A particular example that is valuable to the clinician and often underrated by those who are eager for dramatic radiographs is the *normal* chest radiograph. Only when the normal is known can the abnormal be recognized. Hundreds of normal radiographs should be checked, as well as the abnormalities often encountered in clinical practice. Practice and experience are the next steps needed to become competent in the use of radiographs in patient care.

TABLE OF SELECTED ABNORMALITIES
ON CHEST RADIOGRAPHS

Abnormality	Description	Radiographic Sign	Additional Radiographic Procedures
Pneumothorax	Air within the thoracic cavity, usually within the intrapleural space	Area of radiolucency without tissue markings Clearly demarcated collapsed lung with sharp border of visceral pleura Increased density of collapsed lung In tension pneumothorax, the lung may be compressed against the mediastinum and not be visible, the diaphragm may be flattened or inverted, the intercostal spaces may be widened, the ribs may be more horizontal, and the mediastinum may be shifted to the contralateral side	Chest radiograph taken on full expiration aids in identification of small pneumothorax Follow-up radiographs to check patient's progress
Atelectasis	Absence of gas or air from an area of the lung An area of collapsed lung; the atelectatic area may be very small and not visible on radiographs, as in microatelectasis, or include the entire lung, as would occur with occlusion of a main stem bronchus, which might result from a right main stem intubation	Varies with extent of atelectasis, but frequently includes: Increased density in atelectatic area Shift of mediastinum toward atelectatic area Bowing of interlobar fissures toward atelectasis Elevation of diaphragm on affected side Linear or "platelike" atelectasis appears as linear densities, usually running at right angles to the mediastinum, thought to result from subsegmental collapse With collapse of an entire lung, the intercostal spaces are frequently contracted, in addition to the findings of increased density in the affected hemithorax, deviation of the mediastinum toward the affected side,	Posterior oblique radiograph for lower lobes Lordotic radiograph for right middle lobe Lateral radiograph for left upper lobe

Abnormality	Description	Radiographic Sign	Additional Radiographic Procedures
		and elevation of the dia-phragm on the affected side	
Pneumonia	An inflammatory process of the lungs with multiple etiologies, including bacteria, viruses, fungi and chemical irritants; the inflammatory process frequently involves in-terstitial and exudative changes in the pulmonary parenchyma	The radiographic signs of pneumonia vary con-siderably with the specific etiology; however, there are general signs frequently seen with pneumonia Pneumonia can involve a small area (segmental or subsegmental), a lobe, a lung, or both lungs Pneumonia appears as an area of increased density and may have sharp borders, as in segmental or lobar pneumonia, or have diffuse borders involving several segments and sub-segments The pneumonic area may become consolidated and have an appearance of increasing density on the chest radiograph Air bronchograms can often appear Pneumonic areas may become atelectatic, some-times making it difficult to distinguish atelectasis from pneumonia It is fairly common for pleural effusions to be associated with pneumonia May be difficult to dis-tinguish from pulmonary edema, particularly if both are present	Follow-up radiographs to check patient's progress Lateral decubitus films to determine extent of pneumonia versus pleural effusion
Pulmonary edema —cardiogenic	Accumulation of excess fluid in the interstitium and alveoli, frequently secondary to left ventric-ular failure	May involve areas of one or both lungs Area of increased density, may be perihilar or scattered, often in de-pendent areas Fluffy infiltrates can appear	

138

Abnormality	Description	Radiographic Sign	Additional Radiographic Procedures
		Kerley B lines	Follow-up radiographs to check patient's progress
		Pleural effusion is often evident	
		Often with enlarged cardiac silhouette	
		Diffuse reticular pattern with interstitial edema	
Pulmonary edema— noncardiogenic	Accumulation of excess fluid in the interstitium and alveoli, frequently secondary to damage to the pulmonary capillary endothelium	May be unilateral or bilateral	Follow-up radiographs to check patient's progress
		Area of increased fluffy density, frequently more dense near hilum	
		Pleural effusions are usually *not* present	
		Cardiac silhouette is *not* enlarged	
		Differentiation between cardiogenic and non-cardiogenic pulmonary edema may require pulmonary artery catheter	
COPD— emphysema	Dilation and destruction of airspaces distal to the terminal bronchioles, usually associated with damage to pulmonary vasculature	Emphysema and chronic bronchitis are frequently seen together; on a radiograph, one may note the following:	Fluoroscopy to observe diaphragm movement
		No radiographic abnormality noted in many cases	Ventilation-perfusion scans
		Hyperinflation	
		Diminished lung markings	
		Low, flat diaphragm	
		Long, thin cardiac silhouette	
Chronic bronchitis	Chronic inflammatory process involving the bronchial walls, with mucus gland hypertrophy and increased mucus production	Right ventricle may be enlarged	
		Costal attachments to diaphragm	
		Hyper-radiolucency	
		Enlarged main pulmonary arteries	
		Large retrosternal air space seen in lateral radiograph	

Abnormality	Description	Radiographic Sign	Additional Radiographic Procedures
		Increased A-P diameter	
		Fibrotic changes may be present	
Bronchiectasis	Irreversible dilation of bronchi and bronchioles, often secondary to infection	Chest radiograph may appear normal, if area of bronchiectasis is small	Bronchogram
Cylindrical		Shows dilated bronchial walls without alveoli	
		Cylinder-shaped bronchioles	
		Increased bronchial markings	
		Adjacent emphysema	
		Thickened diaphragmatic pleura	
		Usually involves lower lobes	
Saccular		Large, saclike structures	
		Fibrotic markings	
		Associated atelectasis	
		Adjacent emphysema	
		Thickening of diaphragmatic pleura	
Cystic		Bronchi may be of normal diameter, leading to cysts	
		Cystic areas	
		Adjacent atelectasis	
		Honeycomb appearance	
Pulmonary embolus	Obstruction of pulmonary artery, arteriole or capillaries by blood thrombus, fat globule, etc.	Often no radiographic signs	Pulmonary arteriogram
		Density similar to pneumonia with diffuse borders	Clear termination of affected pulmonary artery on arteriogram
		Hyper-radiolucency distal to embolus caused by decreased perfusion of vasculature	Perfusion scan
		Dilation of pulmonary artery on affected side	

Abnormality	Description	Radiographic Sign	Additional Radiographic Procedures
Pulmonary embolism (cont.)		Pleural effusion on affected side may be evident	
		Ipsilateral hemidiaphragm may be elevated	
		Platelike atelectasis	
		Pulmonary edema, particularly seen with fat embolus	
		Cor pulmonale	
Pleural effusion	Fluid within the intrapleural space may be free or encapsulated (loculated)	An effusion less than 300 mL usually does not show in an upright PA radiograph	Lateral decubitus radiographs to layer out effusion and view lung "behind" the effusion
		Increased density, usually begins at costophrenic angle	Other positions, such as oblique
		Blunting of costophrenic angle with small effusion	
		In PA radiograph, a concave upper border fades into the lung field	Sonograms to determine size and extent of effusion, and to aid in tapping
		In lateral radiograph, the effusion may spread up the anterior and posterior chest wall	
		Interlobar fissures may be highlighted by filling with fluid	
		In large pleural effusion, the entire lung may exhibit whiteout	
		In large pleural effusion, the mediastinum is shifted to the contralateral side, the intercostal spaces become widened, and the ipsilateral hemidiaphragm becomes depressed	
		Loculated effusions may be encapsulated in virtually any intrapleural space	Loculated effusions frequently do not layer out in lateral decubitus radiographs
		Atelectasis may be present	

Abnormality	Description	Radiographic Sign	Additional Radiographic Procedures
Extrapleural lesions	The space between the parietal pleura and the rib cage is the extrapleural space; lesions in this region have several etiologies, including neoplasm and trauma (i.e., hematoma)	Increased uniform density Sharp border facing the lung Tapered edges where the lesions' border meets the chest wall Border is convex toward the lung Pleural effusion is usually absent If rib pathology is the source of the lesion, rib destruction may be present	Multiple projections Tomograms
Cystic fibrosis	Autosomal recessive, inherited disorder of the exocrine glands; in the lung, the mucus-secreting glands secrete viscid mucus that obstructs airways, with secondary infection frequently seen	Bronchial thickening Atelectasis Bronchiectasis Scattered areas of consolidation are frequently more prominent in the upper lung fields Heart may appear narrow, and diaphragms may be flat secondary to airway obstruction and air trapping	Follow-up radiographs to check patient's progress Although not a radiographic procedure, elevated sweat chloride levels are diagnostic

GLOSSARY

angiography—radiographic visualization of blood vessels after injection of radiopaque contrast substance.

AP (anteroposterior) radiograph—a radiograph made in such a manner that the x-ray beam enters from the patient's anterior aspect, exits from the patient's posterior aspect, and then strikes the radiographic film.

arteriogram—radiograph of an artery after injection of a radiopaque substance.

barium—chemical element; barium sulfate is used as a contrast medium in radiography because of its radiopacity.

bronchogram—the visualization of a bronchus in a radiograph; the bronchus may be filled with air or a radiopaque medium.

bulla—a space or vesicle in the lung that is usually greater than 1 cm in diameter.

burned-out—a term meaning overexposure of a radiograph that results in loss of shadows.

cardiac silhouette—outline of the heart projected in the radiograph.

caudal—See directional terms.

cephalad—See directional terms.

coarseness—state of not being fine, not microscopic; a coarse picture would have fewer dots per area to create the image.

consolidation—in the lung, a process whereby the air spaces are filled by a tenacious substance and the lung appears solidified.

contralateral—See directional terms.

costophrenic—pertaining to ribs and diaphragm; the angle formed by ribs and diaphragm.

cutaneous—pertaining to the skin.

density—mass per unit volume; the compactness of a structure or material.

dependent—hanging down.

diffuse—spread out; not concentrated or localized.

Directional terms:

   caudal—toward the tail.

   cephalad—toward the head.

   contralateral—associated with a similar part on the opposite side.

   dorsal—the back or posterior.

   ipsilateral—toward or on the same side.

   lateral—when used as a directional term, away from the center.

   medial—toward the center; opposite of lateral.

   unilateral—affecting or on only one side.

   ventral—the front, abdominal side or anterior.

dorsal—See directional terms.

dosimeter—device, such as a film badge or Geiger counter, that measures radiation exposure.

edema—abnormal accumulation of fluid in tissues or cavities of the body.

exposure—the quantity of radiation that the object of a radiograph was subjected to; this is expressed in mA/s (milliamperes per second).

effusion—excessive fluid in a body cavity; may be transudate or exudate.

fibrosis—replacement of normal tissue with fibrous tissue.

fissure—any narrow cleft or furrow, normal or otherwise.

focal plane—plane of tissue most in focus on a tomogram.

granulation—formation of small grains or particles of tissue, occurring during a healing process.

hemi—prefix meaning one-half; for example, hemidiaphragm.

hilar—pertaining to the hilum.

hilum—in chest radiography, the root of the lungs at the mediastinum, where the vessels, nerves and bronchi enter and exit the lung.

hyperlucent—a structure or material that allows penetration of x-radiation more easily than expected or more easily than a comparative area.

hypolucent—a structure or material that allows penetration of x-radiation less easily than expected or less easily than a comparative area.

ipsilateral—See directional terms.

intercostal—between the ribs.

interstitial—referring to the spaces between tissues.

ion—an atom with a positive or negative charge.

ionization—the process whereby an atom loses or gains electrons to become an ion.

kV(p)—kilovolt peak; the maximum voltage applied to an x-ray-producing tube.

kyphosis—curvature of the spine with the convexity facing backward (posterior).

lateral—See directional terms.

lateral decubitus—a position in which the patient is lying down on one side or the other; in a left lateral decubitus position, the patient would be lying on his left side: the opposite is the case for a right lateral decubitus position.

lateral radiograph—a radiograph taken in which the patient has rotated 90 degrees from the PA or AP position, so that the x-ray beam enters and exits through the patient's sides; in a right lateral radiograph, the film is against the patient's right side and the beam enters from the left side: the opposite is the case for a left lateral radiograph.

lesion—local pathologic change of an organ or body part.

loculated—containing small spaces or cavities.

lordosis—curvature of the spine with the convexity facing forward (anterior).

lordotic position—a position in which the patient stands with his back toward the film and leans back, so that only his shoulders, neck and head touch the film; this can also be done with the patient vertical and the x-ray beam at an angle to view the apices without the superimposed clavicular shadows.

magnification—the enlargement of a body image recorded on the radiograph.

mAs—milliamperes per second; determines the quantity of radiation that is produced.

medial—See directional terms.

mediastinum—space between the pleural sacs of lungs, sternum and thoracic spine; contains the heart and all thoracic viscera, except the lungs.

metastasis—spread of disease from one organ or region to another.

neoplasm—new growth, malignant or benign.

nodule—a small bump or density.

oblique position—a tilted position of the patient in which the x-ray beam enters the patient somewhere in between where it would normally enter for a PA or AP radiograph, and a lateral radiograph; for example, in a left anterior oblique position, the patient's left anterior aspect would be closest to the radiographic film.

PA (posteroanterior) radiograph—a radiograph made in such a manner that the x-ray beam enters from the patient's posterior aspect, exits from the patient's anterior aspect, and then strikes the radiographic film.

penetration—the ability of x-radiation to go into or pass through a substance; the voltage factor.

perfusion scan—technique for obtaining an image of lung perfusion that employs the intravenous injection of a radioisotope (e.g., technetium 99m) and a gamma camera.

position—refers to the specific body position used when the radiograph is taken. The following qualifiers can be used:

1) **anatomical**—subject upright, facing toward the viewer, arms down, palms supinated.

2) **decubitus**—a general term referring to the patient lying down. A lateral decubitus has the patient on the right (right lateral) or left (left lateral) side.

3) **oblique**—the body is turned at approximately a 45 degree angle to the x-ray beam.

4) **prone**—lying on abdomen, horizontally.

5) **recumbent**—lying down in any position (prone, supine, and so on).

6) **supine**—lying on back, horizontally.

7) **Trendelenburg**—lying on back, entire body tilted with head down, feet up.

projection—the path of the x-ray beam upon entering and exiting the body; for example, posteroanterior (PA) means the beam strikes the back first and exits the front before passing through the film.

radiograph—a film record of the image produced when an x-ray beam passes through an object.

radiolucent—a structure or material that allows x-radiation to pass through it without much difficulty; casts little or no shadow on x-ray film.

resolution—the ability to visually distinguish two points from one; a measure of the clarity or sharpness of an image.

reticular—resembling a net; the term "reticulum" means a network.

Roentgen, Wilhelm C.—discovered x-rays in 1895.

roentgen (R)—unit of exposure dose = 2.58 x 10^{-4} coulombs/kg of dry air.

roentgenogram—outdated term for a radiograph.

scoliosis—lateral curvature of the spine.

sharpness—clarity of image; clearly demarcated from surrounding images.

sigh—a large breath, frequently with a volume two to three times the tidal volume.

silhouette sign—the obliteration of a normal silhouette, usually the heart or aorta, by an abnormal thoracic density, such as pneumonia.

spiculated—needlelike in shape or appearance, usually pertaining to a body structure or part.

subcutaneous—beneath the skin.

teleoroentgenography—a radiograph made with the x-ray tube at least six feet from the x-ray film; used to minimize distortion.

tomography—body section radiography; a special radiograph taken at a predetermined depth of a body section.

tortuous—winding, with bends and curves.

tubercle—small nodule or prominence.

unilateral—See directional terms.

ventral—See directional terms.

BIBLIOGRAPHY

Cowan, R.J. "Radionuclide perfusion and ventilation imaging." *Respir Ther* 8 (No. 6) (1978): 14.

Eiken, M. *Roentgen Diagnosis of the Chest.* Chicago: Year Book Medical Publishers, Inc., 1974.

Etter, L.E. *Glossary of Words and Phrases Used in Radiology, Nuclear Medicine and Ultrasound.* 2d ed. Springfield: Charles C. Thomas, Publisher, 1970.

Felson, B. *Chest Roentgenology.* Philadelphia: W.B. Saunders Co., 1973.

Felson, B. "The chest roentgenologic workup—what and why? Conventional methods (Basics of RD)." Reprinted in *Respir Care* 25 (1980): 955.

Felson, B., A.S. Weinstein and H.B. Spitz. *Principles of Chest Roentgenology: A Programmed Text.* Philadelphia: W.B. Saunders Co., 1965.

Fraser, R.G., and J.A.P. Pare. *Organ Physiology: Structure and Function of the Lung with Emphasis on Roentgenology.* 2d ed. Philadelphia: W.B. Saunders Co., 1977.

Jackson, C.L., and J.F. Huber. "Correlated applied anatomy of the bronchial tree and lungs with a system of nomenclature." *Dis Chest* 9 (1943): 319.

Jacob, A., and H.L. Jackson. *Dictionary of Radiologic Terminology.* St. Louis: Warren H. Green, Inc., 1982.

Meschan, I. *Analysis of Roentgen Signs in General Radiology. Volume 2: Respiratory System—Heart.* Philadelphia: W.B. Saunders Co., 1973.

Miller, W.T. "An introduction to chest radiology." *Respir Care* 18 (1973): 304.

Miller, W.T. "Specialized radiographic examinations." *Respir Care* 18 (1973): 452.

Myers, P.A., and T.A. Martin. *Glossary for Radiologic Technologist.* New York: Praeger Publishers, 1981.

Proto, A.V., *et al.* "The chest radiologic workup—special studies." *Respir Care* 26 (1981): 255.

Secker-Walker, R.H., and B.A. Siegel. "The use of nuclear medicine in the diagnosis of lung disease." *Radiol Clin North Am* XI (No. 1) (1973): 215.

Shanks, S.C., and P. Kerley, eds. *A Textbook of X-Ray Diagnosis: Volume III—Respiratory System.* Philadelphia: W.B. Saunders Co., 1973.

Squire, L.F., W.M. Colaiace and N. Strutynsky. *Exercises in Diagnostic Radiology: The Chest.* Philadelphia: W.B. Saunders Co., 1970.

Taplin, G.V., and S.K. Chopra. "Lung perfusion—inhalation scintigraphy in obstructive airway disease and pulmonary embolism." *Radiol Clin North Am* XVI (No. 3) (1978): 491.

SUBJECT INDEX